CANCERS
of the
MOUTH &
THROAT

A PATIENT'S GUIDE TO TREATMENT

William M. Lydiatt, M.D.
Perry J. Johnson, M.D.

Addicus Books
Omaha, Nebraska

An Addicus Nonfiction Book

ISBN 1-886039-44-5
Book design and illustrations by Jack Kusler

This book is not intended to be a substitute for a physician, nor do the authors intend to give advice contrary to that of an attending physician.

Library of Congress Cataloging-in-Publication Data

Lydiatt, William M., 1962.
    Cancers of the mouth & throat : a patient's guide to treatment /William M. Lydiatt, Perry J. Johnson.
        p. cm.
Includes index.
        ISBN 1-886039-44-5
    1. Mouth—Cancer—Popular works. 2. Throat—Cancer—Popular works.
I. Johnson, Perry J., 1964- II. Title.
        RC280.M6 L935 2001
        616.99.431.dc21   00-011134

Addicus Books, Inc.
P.O. Box 45327
Omaha, Nebraska 68145
www.AddicusBooks.com
Printed in the United States of America

10 9 8 7 6

For our patients and their loved ones,
with our profound thanks for teaching us
the meaning of courage, humor, and life.

Contents

Acknowledgments

We would like to acknowledge the work of Dan Lydiatt, D.D.S., M.D., and Ron Hollins, D.M.D., M.D., for laying the foundation of the head and neck cancer program at the University of Nebraska and for providing a model to follow. We have learned a great deal from their example. Many people helped edit the manuscript and offered comments that were used to improve the text, especially Kathy Lydiatt, R.N., Rob Bayer, R.N., Bruce Davidson, M.D., Alan Richards, M.D., Dan Lydiatt, D.D.S., M.D., and Sue Seaman, R.N. Special thanks to Kate Maloy, who helped us clearly present what we wanted to convey, and Rod Colvin and everyone at Addicus Books, who cheerfully provided their insight and experience. We wish to thank Jack Kusler for the illustrations throughout the book. Carol Gable provided insight into swallowing and nutritional disorders. Thanks to Ted Kooser, whose brilliant poetry condenses many complex emotions and thoughts into short, moving pieces of art. We appreciate his allowing us to use his poetry.

I thank my mentors at the University of Nebraska and Memorial Sloan-Kettering Cancer Center, and F. William Karrer at the Nebraska Methodist Hospital, for teaching the technical and humanistic aspects of caring for people with head and neck cancer. Special thanks to my lovely wife, Kathy Lydiatt, R.N., for her expert editorial help in making this manuscript flow with a warmth uniquely hers, and to my children—Max, Joe, and Samantha—for their patience during this process.

Bill Lydiatt

I thank my many mentors at the University of Nebraska and the University of Pittsburgh for their guidance. Special thanks to my wife, Ann, and my children—Taylor, Kaitlin, and Rachael—for their support and encouragement.

Perry Johnson

Introduction

Cancer. Few words convey such potential power, fear, helplessness, anger, and sadness. Virtually all of us have been personally touched by this dreaded disease. It seems everyone has a unique reaction upon hearing this word in association with themselves or a loved one. Because no single cancer behaves exactly the same, part of the fear associated with cancer comes from its unpredictable nature. Nowhere is this more true than with cancers affecting the mouth, throat, voice box, sinuses, thyroid, and salivary glands—collectively known as head and neck cancers. These cancers involve the most basic aspects of our humanity—our ability to speak and eat, even our appearance. Coping with these and other issues are important for all people with head and neck cancer.

This book will help you better understand cancers of the head and throat. With this knowledge you can reduce your anxiety and better deal with the diagnosis and treatment of cancer. The better informed you are, the better questions you can ask, and ultimately the more you can be involved in your treatment. By becoming involved you will feel more in control and take a positive role in your own care.

We do not intend to serve as substitutes for your doctor or other health-care professionals. We do hope you will use this book as a resource whether you have cancer or are caring for someone who does. We have attempted to explain in understandable terms the types of cancers found in the head and neck region, treatment options, treatment side effects and ways to deal with them, and what you might expect as you work through your treatment. We have also tried to stress the importance of one's emotional health after a diagnosis of cancer and its ensuing treatment. By understanding more about this disease, you will be better able to formulate questions for your doctor and take a more active role in your treatment.

We wish you the best in your journey ahead. No single event in your life is likely to have such a profound impact as the diagnosis of cancer. We hope this book will help in some small way to make it a tolerable and even life-affirming experience.

PART I

Understanding Cancers of the Mouth and Throat

At the Cancer Clinic

She is being helped toward the open door
that leads to the examining rooms
by two young women I take to be her sisters.
Each bends to the weight of an arm
and steps with the straight, tough bearing
of courage. At what must seem to be
a great distance, a nurse holds the door,
smiling and calling encouragement.
How patient she is in the crisp white sails
of her clothes. The sick woman
peers from under her funny knit cap
to watch each foot swing scuffing forward
and take its turn under her weight.
There is no restlessness or impatience
or anger anywhere in sight. Grace
fills the clean mold of this moment
and all the shuffling magazines grow still.

—*Ted Kooser*
Poet Laureate
of the United States
(2004-2005)

1

Cancers of the Mouth and Throat

If you have cancer, you are not alone. Each year, nearly 50,000 Americans develop a cancer of the lip, mouth, tongue, tonsils, throat, larynx, salivary glands, nose, and sinuses. Nearly 75 percent of these new cases are men. The incidence of mouth and throat cancer among women is, however, on the rise. As many as 500,000 are survivors of these cancers.

What Is Cancer?

Cancer is a group of cells growing out of control. Let's take a closer look at how this process occurs. Our cells contain a complicated set of instructions called DNA. These instructions tell a cell how to perform its job—that is, how to be a skin cell, a brain cell, a liver cell, and so on. They also tell the cell when to reproduce and when to die. DNA is the major constituent of our *chromosomes*, which determine what species we are and also what our individual traits will be, from our height and hair color to many aspects of our personality. Thus ,DNA is often called the "building block" of life.

Sometimes, though, DNA can tear down what it has built. If a cell's DNA is damaged—for example, by a virus or toxic substance—the cell will usually die. Occasionally, instead, the abnormal cell will begin reproducing rapidly, creating ever greater numbers of new cells that also carry the DNA damage.

The more abnormal a cell's DNA becomes, the more abnormally the cell will behave. In turn, this increasingly abnormal behavior creates more and more mistakes within

1

Normal Cells

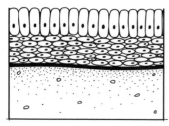

Cells are similar in shape and grow in an orderly manner. Cells are aligned and the tops of the cells are flat.

Precancerous Cells

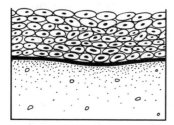

Dysphasia. The cells and their nuclei become irregular and misshapen. The basement membrane remains intact.

Cancer

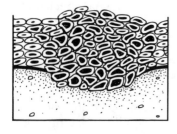

Early cancer. Cancer cells now break through the basement membrane. This "invasion" is typical of cancer.

the cell. These DNA "mistakes"are called *mutations.* It appears that damaged cells must have between six and ten different mistakes before they begin behaving like a cancer.

Take, for example, the cells that make up the mucous membrane of the mouth and throat. These cells normally divide and reproduce only when old cells die or other cells are scraped away in normal activities such as chewing and swallowing. Under strict DNA instructions, the cells next to those that have died or been scraped away will reproduce to replace them. Once the dead cells have been replaced, the process of cell replication stops.

However, if the cells are exposed to excessive tobacco smoke, alcohol, or other hazards, their DNA may be damaged. They may pass the damage on to the next generation of cells as they reproduce. As larger and larger generations of abnormal cells are formed, they may eventually become visible as white or red patches in the mouth or throat. These are known as *precancerous lesions.* With time, the lesions may increase in both size and abnormality until they finally become true cancers.

Unfortunately, the out-of-control cell growth that causes

cancer does not usually stop with the formation of a single tumor. Instead, the abnormal cells tend to invade surrounding tissue and can spread even farther, through the blood or through the lymphatic system. The lymphatic system includes channels, similar to veins, that carry white blood cells and nutrients and drain waste products away from tissues and cells. These channels contain rounded masses of tissue called *lymph nodes*, which filter bacteria, viruses, and cancer cells out of the lymphatic fluid.

When cancer spreads beyond the place where the first abnormal cells develop, each resulting new cancer is called a *metastasis*. When a group of cells grows into a mass that does not invade or spread elsewhere, the mass is called a *benign*— that is, a noncancerous—*tumor*, and it has a much better prognosis than cancer.

Health professionals also speak of cancers in terms of "grade". The higher the grade, the more aggressive the cancer and the likelihood that the cancer will come back after treatment. Lymph node involvement is also more likely in high-grade than low-grade tumors. High-grade cancers are more likely to spread to other areas of the body.

Causes of Mouth and Throat Cancer

Tobacco

Smoking cigarettes, or chewing or sniffing tobacco can put a person at high risk for cancer. All forms of tobacco are dangerous, but cigarette smoke is probably the most dangerous. Most people automatically think of lung cancer when they think of the risks of smoking, but cancer can form at any site that has contact with tobacco or its by-products. In fact, 90 percent of people with mouth and throat cancer have been users of tobacco in some form.

The tissues of the mouth and throat are directly exposed to harmful chemicals in tobacco, including formaldehyde, benzo-a-pyrene, nitrogen oxides, urethane, nickel, cadmium, radioactive polonium, hydrazine, and nitrosodiethylamine. These are known to damage the DNA in the cells at the site of contact.

Tobacco products can also damage other areas of the body, including the sinuses, esophagus, salivary glands, lungs, even the kidneys and bladder. All these tend to be sensitive to the effects of tobacco. Damage to these more distant parts of the body occurs after special proteins called *enzymes* have broken down the chemicals in tobacco. These enzymes reduce harmful substances to much smaller components that can be excreted through the urine. However, the broken-down products of tobacco can themselves be harmful. When the kidneys and bladder, for example, come into contact with these products, cellular damage can occur in those areas as well as in the mouth or throat.

Still, not everyone who uses tobacco will develop cancer, and some who have never used it will. In general, however, tobacco use is the biggest known cause of cancers of the mouth and throat. In fact, smoking 1 to 2 packs of cigarettes a day for 20 years or more gives you a risk of mouth or throat cancer that is 2 to 8 times greater than that of a nonsmoker. The more you smoke, the higher your risk. Women have a higher risk than men who smoke the same amount. One pack of cigarettes a day for a woman is roughly equivalent to 1.25 packs for a man.

Alcohol

Alcohol in large quantities (more than five drinks per day for men and somewhat fewer for women) is known to increase the risk of mouth and throat cancers—especially those at the floor of the mouth, base of the tongue, tonsils, and lower pharynx. As many as 80 percent of people with these cancers use alcohol regularly. Heavy drinking (five or more drinks per day) alone creates a risk that is five to eight times greater than that of a nondrinker. The combination of heavy alcohol use and tobacco use is particularly dangerous. For example, a person who consumes two packs of cigarettes and five drinks each day is about forty times more likely to get cancer than someone who does not smoke or drink. Hard liquor is probably riskier than beer, which is riskier than wine.

Other Toxins

Overexposure to any of countless chemicals and hazardous substances can predispose people to a variety of cancers. Mouth and throat cancers have been linked, in particular, to mustard gas, wood dust, cadmium, leather manufacturing, isopropyl alcohol manufacturing, nickel, and chewing betel nut, a common practice in India.

Exposure to sunlight is also well known to increase the risk of skin cancers and lip cancer as well. Serious sunburns in childhood create risk for adult skin cancers. People with light skin and freckles, especially those of northern European descent, are at highest risk. It is important to use sun protection. Clothing that blocks the sun is best, since the use of sun-blocking creams is controversial. Some recent studies suggest the creams might actually raise the risk of sun damage, perhaps by giving users a false sense of security that prompts them to stay out in the sun longer. Other studies show a positive effect. Overall, the use of sun-blocking agents is probably better than no sunblock.

Severe stomach acid reflux can also elevate the risk of cancers of the esophagus and the lower throat. Exposure to radiation as a child creates a risk for cancer later, as an adult. A virus, human papilloma virus, has also been linked to some cancers of the throat.

Heredity

Although some cancers appear to run in some families, cancers of the mouth and throat tend to be inherited only through rare genetic syndromes.

- *Li-Fraumeni syndrome* is a mutation of a special gene that makes a protein necessary for repairing cellular damage. The mutation inhibits the repair process and therefore raises the risk of cancer.
- *Bloom's syndrome* is associated with short stature, increased sun sensitivity, immune deficiency, and a higher risk of mouth cancer, especially of the lip and tongue.
- *Fanconi's anemia* is associated with abnormal skin pigmentation, growth retardation, and blood abnor-

malities such as anemia, and this too carries an increased risk of mouth cancer.

- *Xeroderma pigmentosum* involves extreme sensitivity to sunlight and puts affected individuals at a much higher risk for lip and skin cancers.

If you or any of your relatives have any of these syndromes, or if members of your family have had cancer, ask your doctor about your degree of risk. He or she might advise you to talk with a genetics counselor, who could help assess whether you or your family members may be at particular risk.

Areas of the Mouth and Throat Affected by Cancer

Mouth

The mouth includes the lips, gums, teeth, tongue, hard palate (roof of the mouth), floor of the mouth, and inner cheeks. Each of these components plays a major role in the quality and sustenance of life. If any one of them is compromised by disease, it can threaten a person's ability to breathe, eat, or speak.

Throat

The throat aids in swallowing, allows the passage of breath, and produces sound. The tubelike pharynx handles swallowing. The muscles of the pharynx squeeze food down to the esophagus, a larger tubelike structure that takes over the job until the food reaches the stomach. The larynx, which is connected to the trachea (windpipe) and is actually part of the respiratory system, handles sound and breath.

Pharynx

The pharynx, or throat, is composed of the *oropharynx, nasopharynx,* and *hypopharynx.* "Oro" is Latin for mouth, and "pharynx" is derived from the Greek word for throat. Thus the oropharynx ("mouth-throat") begins at the back of the mouth and includes the tonsils, soft palate, *uvula* (that bit of tissue that hangs down at the back of your throat), and base (rearmost part) of the tongue. The *nasopharynx* ("nose-throat") is a very

Mouth and Throat Side View

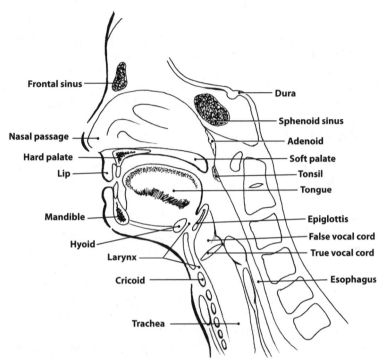

small area above the soft palate and behind the nose. It contains the *adenoids*, small masses of infection-fighting tissue that are part of the lymphatic system. The *eustachian tube* connects the middle ear to the nasopharynx. When fluids accumulate in the middle ear as a result of illness or infection, the eustachian tube may become swollen or blocked. The eustachian tube also produces the "pop"in your ears when you experience a change in altitude or air pressure. The *hypopharynx* ("underthroat") is difficult to see without special equipment. Located behind the larynx, it connects the pharynx to the esophagus.

Larynx

The larynx, or voice box, is located in front of the pharynx and just below the back of the tongue. It can be felt in the neck as the Adam's apple. It has three compartments—the *glottis*, *supraglottis*, and *subglottis*.

The glottis is formed by the *vocal cords,* which tighten and loosen to produce sounds of varying pitch. The tongue, cheeks, teeth, and lips then shape the sounds into words. Pitch variation is an important, expressive aspect of speech but a minor requirement for basic communication.

The supraglottis, or top portion of the larynx, consists of a flap of cartilage called the *epiglottis* and other structures called *false vocal cords,* which we use for whispering. Together, these structures shunt food and liquids backward, away from the trachea and into the pharynx. This protects against choking and keeps food and liquids out of the lungs.

The subglottis is the space below the true vocal cords and just above the trachea.

Sinuses

The *paranasal sinuses,* located behind and beside the base of the nose, are air-filled cavities in the skull. They are lined with mucous membranes. Sinuses play an important role in speech—the sound made by your larynx and throat resonates in your sinuses, making your voice audible and giving it your characteristic sound. When you get a cold, your sinuses get congested and the membranes swell, giving the sound of your voice a nasal quality. The four major sinuses in your head are the *frontal, maxillary, ethmoid,* and *sphenoid sinuses.*

The frontal sinus, located above your eyes and behind your forehead, does not develop until adolescence. It determines the shape of your adult forehead, and the thick bones surrounding it protect your brain from injury. Tumors usually do not affect this sinus.

The sinuses most susceptible to tumors are the maxillary and ethmoid sinuses. The maxillary sinuses, located under your eyes, help form the floor of your eye sockets. They are the sinuses most frequently affected by sinus infections. Nerves that supply sensation to the middle part of your face and your top teeth run through this sinus. A tumor involving these nerves can create numbness or tingling of the face or upper teeth. Surgical removal of this sinus can also cause numbness in these areas. The ethmoid sinuses, containing nerves that create your sense of smell, are located between your eyes.

The bones that separate the sinuses are eggshell thin;

Paranasal Sinuses

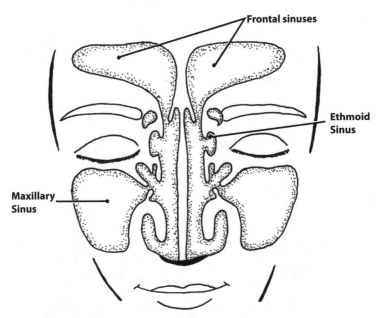

however, they can play an important role in acting as a barrier to the spread of cancer. One such bone is the *cribriform plate*, located right on top of the ethmoid sinuses. This bone has many perforations through which the nerves for the sense of smell pass from the nose to the brain and back. Also, the *dura*, a thick covering of tissue, surrounds the brain and further inhibits the invasion of cancer cells. Still another barrier is the *periorbita*, the thick lining of the eye sockets which protects the eyeballs from the spread of a tumor.

The sphenoid sinus is situated almost in the center of your head. It is surrounded by the nasopharynx below, the brain on the top and three sides, and the nasal cavity in the front. It is the least common site for sinus tumors.

Salivary Glands

These glands produce *saliva*, which lubricates food for swallowing and contains special proteins called enzymes that begin the digestive process. There are three pairs of major salivary glands—the *parotid, submandibular,* and *sublingual*

9

Neck Lymph Nodes

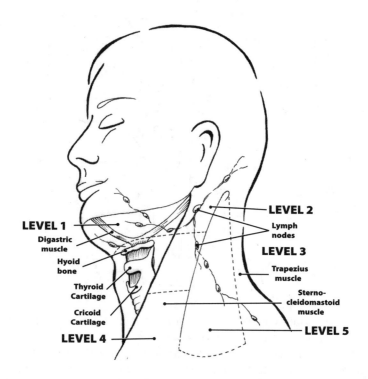

Lymph nodes in the neck are divided into five regions, shown above as levels. The lymph nodes, approximately 200 total, are located under the sternocleidomastoid muscle.

glands. The largest of these are the parotid ("around the ear") glands, located on each cheek, just in front of the ear and overlying part of the jawbone. The submandibular ("under jaw") glands are partially under each side of the lower jawbone. The sublingual ("under tongue") glands are inside the jawbone and under each side of the tongue.

There are also between 600 and 1,000 minor salivary glands within the mucous membranes that line your tongue, lips, palate, throat, nose, and sinuses. These glands cannot be seen without a microscope.

Neck

The neck contains nerves that permit most of the activities of the mouth and throat, including the nerves to the tongue, larynx, and pharynx. If cancer invades any of these nerves, it usually destroys or damages their function. For example, if the major nerve to the tongue is invaded, you will notice a slurring of speech, and if the nerve to the vocal cord is invaded, you will become hoarse.

The neck also contains the lymph nodes, the first areas to which mouth and throat cancers generally spread. The lymph nodes are small, bean-shaped glands that filter out bacteria, viruses, and cancer cells. They swell if they become infected or cancerous.

Types of Mouth and Throat Cancer

The type of a cancer is determined by its cell of origin. That is, where did the cancer start—in cells of the skin, fatty tissue, muscle, cartilage, or bone? Certain areas of the mouth and throat are more prone to cancers because they come into contact with cancer-causing substances. Determining the precise type of a cancer is important since treatment will be based on the type of cancer present.

Carcinomas

Squamous Cell Carcinoma

Squamous means "flat." The tough, protective squamous cells make up the skin and also the mucous membranes inside the mouth and throat. Cancers that begin in these cells— squamous cell carcinomas—represent more than 90 percent of all cancers of the mouth and throat. They are usually caused by tobacco use. They are also one of the most common skin cancers.

Salivary Gland Tumors

More than 75 percent of tumors of the salivary glands occur in the parotid glands. Fortunately, most are benign. Tumors in the submandibular glands account for about 10 to 15 percent of salivary gland tumors, but only about half of these are benign. The remaining salivary gland tumors, which occur in the sublingual and minor glands, are more often malignant. Because salivary glands contain many different types of cells, different types of cancers can arise in them. However, most are carcinomas.

Mucoepidermoid Carcinoma

This is the most common salivary gland cancer. It can form in any of the salivary glands but is seen most often in the parotid glands. Mucoepidermoid carcinomas are categorized as low, intermediate, or high-grade cancers based on their microscopic characteristics.

Adenoid Cystic Carcinoma

This is the most common cancer of the minor and sublingual salivary glands, and possibly of the submandibular glands as well. These tumors tend to grow slowly, tracking along nerves.

The weakness of a nerve, particularly a facial weakness, may indicate the presence of a tumor. These tumors can be extremely persistent, recurring many years after treatment. They are less likely to spread to lymph nodes but many times will spread to the lungs, liver, or bones. Close, ongoing follow-up is very important.

Adenocarcinoma

Adenocarcinomas arise either from minor salivary glands or from the small glands that make up the major salivary glands. Like squamous cell carcinomas, they can spread to the lymph nodes, lungs, or other organs.

Lymphoepithelial Cancer

This cancer occurs in the tonsils, adenoids, or at the base of the tongue, where lymph tissue is commonly found. It tends to spread to lymph nodes very early and will often show up as a neck mass with a very small primary tumor in the tonsil or nasopharynx. These small tumors are found only after careful searching.

This is the most common cancer affecting people of Asian descent and by far the most common tumor of the nasopharynx worldwide. Lymphoepithelial cancer is associated with the Epstein-Barr virus, a common cause of upper respiratory infections. The vast majority of people infected by this virus will not develop cancer, but it does seem to be associated with a high number of these cancers. Lymphoepithelial cancer is also associated with certain risk factors, including poor ventilation and a diet heavy in salted fish.

Sarcomas

These cancers can develop from the cells of muscle, fat, bone, connective tissue, or cartilage almost anywhere in the body. They are categorized either as high-grade or low-grade cancers, which helps predict their behavior and prognosis.

There are many types of sarcoma. The treatment for each depends on the site where it first arises. For example, an *osteosarcoma* may start in the bone of the mandible or upper jaw. *Rhabdomyosarcoma* begins in the muscles. This tumor is often seen in children. The most common sarcoma in adults, *malignant fibrous histiocytoma*, arises in the soft tissues of the head and neck. The prognosis for all sarcomas tends to depend on their size and grade. The smaller the tumor and the lower the grade, the better the prognosis.

Neuroendocrine Cancer

Melanoma

These cancers form in the cells that make pigment when they are exposed to sunlight—the cells that give you a tan. They usually occur on the skin but can also be found in all areas of the mouth and throat. The more deeply the abnormal forms of these cells invade the affected tissue, the more aggressive the cancer will be.

Esthesioneuroblastoma

This cancer begins in the olfactory nerves, which give you your sense of smell. This tumor can occur at any age and, in fact, is often seen in young people.

Lymphomas

Lymphomas begin in the lymph system and can occur anywhere that lymph tissue is found. The term does not refer to cancers that have originated elsewhere and spread to the lymph nodes.

Lymphomas can involve lymph nodes in one area only or throughout the entire body, including the liver, spleen, bone marrow, and even the skin. The head and neck region alone has about 200 lymph nodes. Lymphomas often arise in the neck but can also form in the tonsils, adenoids, tongue, mouth, and throat.

2

Getting a Diagnosis

Getting a diagnosis—confirming whether or not you have cancer—can be a frightening proposition. The time one waits for various test results is stressful, to say the least. Many patients describe it as being on an "emotional roller coaster." But rest assured, cancers of the mouth and throat are among the most curable cancers if they are caught early. The survival rate for these cancers five years after diagnosis is 50 percent, which is very high. With cancers of the tongue or larynx, the rate is even higher—60 percent overall, and 90 percent if detected early.

Accordingly, it is important to get a diagnosis as soon as possible. Fortunately, with cancers of the mouth and throat, early detection is common. Why? The symptoms—impaired tongue movement, persistent hoarseness, a lump in the mouth or throat—tend to be obvious and prompt individuals to see a physician. If you even suspect that a change you have noticed in your body or its functions could indicate cancer, you should see a doctor without delay.

Warning Signs and Symptoms

The following symptoms should be evaluated by a physician if they persist longer than two weeks, progressively worsen, or occur on only one side of the body. In come cases, you might be referred to a specialist.

Hoarseness

Persistent hoarseness is one of the most common signs of cancer of the vocal cords and larynx. Sometimes it arises along with a cough, blood in the phlegm, increasingly noisy breathing, or progressive difficulty in breathing.

Sore Throat, Mouth Sore, or Lesion

A sore throat or a mouth sore that does not go away in a week or two can be a sign of throat or mouth cancer. White or red patches on the skin of the throat or mouth may be precancerous conditions known as *leukoplakia* or *erythroplasia*. They can be treated to prevent a cancer from forming. There are almost no symptoms associated with these precancerous conditions, and only a visual inspection can detect them. This is why routine evaluations by your doctor or dentist are important.

Lump in the Mouth, Throat, Neck, or Cheek

Many cancers have only one symptom at first—a lump, which is often painless. This is especially true of throat cancers and salivary gland cancers. Occasionally, people discover a mouth cancer when a lump interferes with the fit of their dentures. Any new lump should be seen by a doctor. This becomes urgent if the lump is more than half an inch in diameter, is hard and growing, and/or is located in an area where cancers are especially prone to arise. Some of these lumps will be benign tumors or will be caused by infection. Lumps that are soft are rarely cancerous. Still, any new lump should be evaluated.

Change in Speech Quality

Progressive changes in speech—especially a growing inability to speak clearly or an increasingly muffled quality to your voice—could indicate tongue or throat cancer. Over time, tongue cancer can deprive a person of any ability to enunciate because it can completely restrict tongue movement. Any of the symptoms affecting speech can be accompanied by bad breath, so that, too, can be considered a possible warning sign.

Difficulty Swallowing

Cancer of the throat—either the pharynx or esophagus—can gradually make swallowing difficult. If heavier, solid foods like meat become hard to swallow at first, with lighter, softer foods and liquids increasingly presenting a problem, that could mean that a tumor is gradually narrowing the esophagus. Cancer of the pharynx may also result in a feeling that food is catching in the throat. If the lower pharynx is involved, food may get into the trachea. This is known as *aspiration*, and it generally causes coughing while eating.

Nosebleeds

If you experience recurrent nosebleeds, or if your nose is constantly plugged on one side only, you should see your doctor. These can be symptoms of a sinus or nasopharyngeal cancer blocking the nasal passage. With trauma or blowing of the nose, the tumor can crack and bleed through the nose. Most nosebleeds are caused simply by dry air and a deviated septum—a deviation or injury to the cartilage "wall" inside the center of the nose. Other common causes include exposure to wood dust, chemicals, or other irritants. People with a long history of nosebleeds are no more susceptible to cancer than anyone else. But nosebleeds that develop suddenly should always be investigated.

Hearing Loss and Earache

Normal hearing loss associated with aging usually occurs in both ears at about the same rate. But, if you have persistent hearing loss or a sense of fullness in one ear, or pain that is always on the same side, this may be the first sign of a tumor of the nasopharynx. Similarly, though fluid in the middle ear is common and nearly always benign in children, in adults it, too, can indicate a tumor.

If there is no obvious cause of earache or fullness—such as allergy, viral infections, or altitude changes—the nasopharynx should be examined to rule out the possibility of a tumor blocking the eustachian tube. The examination is performed with an instrument called a *nasal endoscope*, which allows your doctor to examine the back of your nasal passages.

In general, any earache that does not go away should be evaluated by your doctor. If the ear itself is found to be normal, with no infection, he or she will examine your throat. Persistent pain in the ear can be "referred" pain from an irritated nerve lower in the throat. Such pain can be created when a cancer of the throat has invaded a nerve that supplies sensation to the ear. The pain is often intensified by the act of swallowing and can be made even worse by eating hot or spicy foods. Referred pain is usually described as deep, penetrating, or just under the ear. It is usually caused by infection or acid reflux, but it should always be evaluated.

Facial Numbness, Asymmetry, or Changes in Eyesight
Tumors of the sinuses can damage or destroy nerves that supply sensation to the lips and cheeks. If you notice a loss of sensation in these areas, especially if you also have a lump or a change in your eyesight, you need to be examined. Your symptoms could be caused by a tumor of the maxillary sinus, which can push into the eye socket and put pressure on the eyeball, resulting in double vision, asymmetry or fullness of the cheek, or numbness of the cheek.

Choosing a Doctor
If you are worried about any of the symptoms listed above, your best first step is to ask your family doctor to evaluate you or refer you to a specialist. The latter may be an ear, nose, and throat (ENT) specialist or an oral surgeon, depending on where the trouble is. If you don't have a regular doctor, call your local cancer center, hospital, or university medical center for options.

Once you have found an appropriate physician to evaluate your symptoms, he/she will review your medical history, discuss with you the history of your symptoms, and examine you. These steps will determine which tests come next. The following guide will help you understand what happens during this first visit to the doctor.

Medical History

Your medical history is likely to give your doctor a good deal of information about your susceptibility to particular kinds of cancer. You will be asked how and when you first noticed the problem, and how it affects your life. Your doctor will also ask you about symptoms—when they started, how long they have been present, and whether they are getting worse. Identifying the body parts that are affected helps to predict what kind of cancer might be present. For example, a lump that has been present for ten years with no change is not likely to be cancerous.

On the other hand, a lump in the mouth that you first noticed six weeks ago, one that has grown larger and has started to affect your speech, would be of concern. Similarly, a lump in the neck that is growing and is accompanied by an earache on the same side is worrisome. Generally, symptoms that have been present for several weeks to months, especially if they are getting worse, are the ones that cause the greatest concern.

During your initial examination, your doctor will also ask you about your exposure to known cancer-causing agents such as tobacco and alcohol. He or she will ask about your general health, any medications you are taking, and whether you are having any other health problems. This is important for several reasons. It will give your doctor a better idea of how much at risk you are for cancer and whether your symptoms might be medications that can cause side effects such as mouth sores, plugged ears, or various kinds of pain.

Your doctor will probably ask you detailed questions about all aspects of your life. These might make you uncomfortable at first, but they are *not* meant to invade your privacy. In fact, if your doctor does not question you closely, he or she might miss opportunities to help you in important ways.

Physical Examination

During your physical examination, your doctor will examine your ears, nose, throat, and mouth. He/she will also check for lumps in your neck, cheeks, and thyroid gland. The doctor will use a mirror to look at your larynx and upper throat. This could make you gag a little, but it does not hurt.

If a more detailed examination of your nasal passages or larynx is required, the doctor will use either a flexible or a rigid scope, inserting it after applying a topical anesthetic to numb your nose. The anesthetic does not taste good, but it eases discomfort involved in inserting the scope, which takes only a minute or two. Your doctor will then ask you to say "e," which makes your vocal cords move and identifies any abnormalities in the function of the larynx. The scope gives your doctor an excellent view of the nasal passages and larynx, along with any lumps or ulcers that are otherwise hard to see.

Altogether, your medical history review, symptom review, and physical examination will take fifteen to thirty minutes. Some of the information will be gathered in advance by the nurse or by a questionnaire given to you in the waiting room. Make sure to answer all questions completely and truthfully. This saves time and allows you to think about any symptoms you might not have mentioned, perhaps thinking they were not relevant or not very serious. Together, the questionnaire and examination will give your doctor enough information to develop a plan, which could require tests such as those described below.

Biopsy

If your physical examination turns up a lump or ulceration, the next step is likely a *biopsy.* In this procedure a small sample of affected tissue is removed and then sent to a laboratory to be analyzed for cancer cells. Sometimes the tissue sample can be taken in the doctor's office—as in the case of visible sores in the mouth. Sometimes, the biopsy requires admission to the hospital or a visit to an outpatient clinic. During an office procedure, the sore or other affected site is numbed, and a small piece of tissue is cut out and sent out for analysis.

Certain suspicious lumps—for example, in the neck or salivary glands—can be biopsied in the doctor's office using a procedure called *fine needle aspiration (FNA).* In this case, your doctor can insert a very narrow needle to withdraw a sample of cells directly from the lump. Sometimes the area is numbed, and sometimes it is not, depending on your own and your doctor's preference. Usually, it takes two aspirations to get enough cells for a diagnosis.

In other cases, when a biopsy cannot be taken easily in the office, your doctor may recommend that it be carried out under general anesthesia. This is standard procedure for areas like the throat and larynx, which are not as accessible as the mouth or neck. This kind of biopsy, usually performed on an outpatient basis, requires a special scope. This scope allows biopsy forceps to be inserted through it. You will very likely go home the same day the biopsy is performed.

If your symptoms suggest that you might have cancer in more than one location, your doctor might also look at your lungs or esophagus during a biopsy of throat or larynx tissue. While you are under anesthesia, he or she can feel any tumor or lesion to determine the extent of the disease without causing you pain.

Regardless of how a biopsy is performed, once the tissue sample is in the laboratory, a *pathologist* (a doctor who specializes in interpreting cell changes caused by disease) will examine the specimen under the microscope. If cancerous cells are detected, the pathologist will determine which type of cancer is present and will inform your doctor. If the initial biopsy doesn't yield enough information for an exact diagnosis, further biopsies will be needed. Biopsy results are usually back in one to five days.

Imaging

Imaging, the general term for X-rays and body scans, is not always necessary but can often be very useful. A special X-ray—a *panorex X-ray*—can show the jaw and teeth in good detail and can often detect whether cancer has invaded the bone. Otherwise, X-rays do not provide sufficient detail to evaluate masses in the mouth or throat. However, there are several other ways of obtaining clear images of a suspicious lump or lesion that can't be seen directly.

CT Scan

Called a *computed tomography*, or a *CT scan*, this technique gives remarkable detail, showing not only what a suspicious lump looks like but how it affects surrounding tissues and whether other lumps or lymph nodes are abnormal. A CT scan requires that you lie on a table while a tubelike machine, which surrounds your body, moves over the area being examined. Usually, a CT scan involves the injection of a special contrasting agent, given through a vein, which highlights physical structures such as blood vessels so that all parts of the image can easily be distinguished. The contrast feels hot when it goes into your vein. If you have a known allergy to contrast, are allergic to iodine, or have any kidney problems, tell your doctor. Allergic reactions to the CT contrast are uncommon, but in cases where they might occur, either the contrast will not be used or medications or fluid will be given before the CT to minimize any ill effects. The test takes about ten to twenty minutes to administer, depending on how many areas are being examined.

MRI

Magnetic resonance imaging (MRI) is similar to a CT scan but takes a little longer to do. The tube used to obtain the image is also narrower, so it feels closer around the body. The MRI is better at examining soft tissues, especially the brain, than the CT scan. A different contrasting agent is used in MRI, and allergic reactions are rare.

Ultrasound

Ultrasound, another imaging technique, is the same painless procedure used to examine a forming baby in the womb. However, it does not provide nearly as much detail as other methods, especially with respect to bone. It is used most often to evaluate thyroid and certain neck masses. Once in a while, ultrasound is used to help a doctor guide a needle during a biopsy.

PET Scan

Finally, *positron-emission tomography*—a *PET scan*— is often used to detect cancer in various parts of the body. However, its use in pretreatment planning is not yet standard for mouth or throat cancer because its reliability for those areas has not yet been proven. PET scans rely on a sugar contrasting agent taken orally. In PET scans, the agent shows cellular activity, especially areas of increased metabolism. Cancer cells, which thrive on sugar, show up as bright areas on the scan.

Team Approach

Depending on the results of your evaluation—your medical history, physical examination, and biopsy—you may be referred to a specialist, or even a team of specialists, for your definitive care.

To better understand the team approach, take the example of a mouth cancer that has spread to a portion of the tongue and jawbone (mandible). Your doctors must determine which kind of therapy will give you the best results with the fewest complications. The decision may involve a surgeon who specializes in mouth and throat cancers, a plastic surgeon, a radiation oncologist, a specialist in chemotherapy, and perhaps a radiologist (a specialist in imaging techniques), and a pathologist. If your doctors recommend radiation in or near your mouth, you will also need to be seen by a dental specialist to evaluate potential damages to your teeth. After treatment, you might need the services of a speech therapist.

Usually, the head and neck surgeon will head up your team. The team leader will serve as your primary contact during both treatment and follow-up. Your primary doctor, or family physician, will continue to serve as the point person for your overall health care.

It is also important to stress that it is perfectly reasonable for a patient to seek a second opinion if he/she has any doubts about a diagnosis or if questions are unanswered. Sometimes, patients don't realize that, especially when the diagnosis is serious, many patients will seek second opinions. Physicians do not find this practice unusual.

How Soon Does Treatment Start?

As you look toward treatment, keep in mind treatment for these cancers is considered urgent, but not an emergency. Accordingly, a general time frame for having surgery or beginning other treatment is one to four weeks after diagnosis. This time frame is reasonable, given the relatively moderate growth rate of squamous cell carcinomas.

3

Staging Cancer

As soon as a cancer diagnosis is confirmed, the next step is to determine how advanced the disease is and whether it has spread from its original site. This is called staging the cancer, and knowing the stage of the cancer is essential in determining the most effective treatment.

Staging Squamous Cell Carcinoma

The standard method of staging mouth and throat cancers is the *TNM system*. It documents the stage of the disease according to the size and extent of the original tumor and whether it has spread to other parts of the body. This universal system tells any health-care professional involved with your case how extensive your cancer is. It stages squamous cell carcinoma very well, and most mouth and throat cancers are of this type. Other types of cancers, including lymphoma and sarcoma, are staged slightly differently, since they behave differently than squamous cell carcinoma.

T: Size or Extent of Tumor

Each component of the TNM system is measured on a scale of 0 to 4. The "T" refers to a tumor's size or extent. Extent refers to how much of the original site a tumor has invaded and whether it interferes with normal body function at that site. The T measurement starts at 1 for the smallest tumors and for those that impair function the least or affect the smallest area.

Some tumors are given a T score according to size, others according to extent. For example, tumors of the mouth, oropharynx, and salivary glands are easy to see and to examine physically, so they are graded only by size, from T1 for the smallest to T4 for the largest. Tumors that are located in areas that are difficult to see or feel are graded by extent rather than size. These include tumors of the larynx, hypopharynx, nasopharynx, and paranasal sinuses. In these cases, T1 indicates the least extensive (or invasive) tumors—those that affect only a part of the original site and do not interfere significantly with body function. A somewhat more extensive tumor (one that involves all or most of the original site and *either* extends to an adjacent site *or* noticeably impedes function) is a T2. It becomes a T3 if it has invaded the entire original site and involves additional surrounding sites or significantly hampers normal function (for example, by paralyzing a vocal cord). As soon as it moves aggressively into nearby major structures (such as the brain, in cancers of the paranasal sinuses and nasopharynx; or the thyroid cartilage, in cancers of the larynx or hypopharynx) it becomes a T4.

N: Lymph Node Involvement

The N-score in the cancer classification refers only to the lymph nodes nearest the primary site. These are the areas to which a cancer is most likely to begin spreading. In the case of mouth and throat cancers, the nearest lymph nodes are in the neck. If other lymph nodes elsewhere in the body are affected by the cancer, that represents a metastasis and is reflected in the M score.

An N score is determined by the number and size of affected lymph nodes found in the neck. The larger the number of affected nodes, and the larger the individual nodes, the greater the degree of involvement. A score of N0 generally indicates that no cancer has been detected in any of the nodes. The N score rises from 1 through 3 as more and larger cancerous nodes are discovered.

When physical examination locates lymph nodes that are larger or harder than normal, it is often difficult to tell for sure whether tumors are present or the nodes are infected by a bacterium or virus or whether cancer is present. Sometimes a biopsy is required for a firm diagnosis.

M: Spread to Other Body Sites

The "M" stands for metastasis, the spread of the cancer to other tissues, bones, or organs such as the lungs or liver. The presence of spreading cancer is suggested by blood tests or imaging techniques and confirmed by a biopsy and tissue analysis. If the cancer has not spread beyond the original site or the lymph nodes, it is designated M0. If it has spread, it is classified as M1.

Overall Stage

Once a score has been assigned to each of the three TNM components, the scores are combined to tell physicians which overall stage the cancer has reached—stage I, II, III, or IV. For example, an overall score of T1N0M0 would indicate that your tumor is of the smallest size or extent (T1), that it does not involve the lymph nodes (N0), and that it has not spread to other parts of the body (M0). This is a stage I cancer. Here is a general description of the stages:

- Stage I cancer is small and found only in the original site.
- Stage II cancer is slightly larger or more extensive but has not spread to the nearby lymph nodes or elsewhere in the body.
- Stage III cancer is characterized by one relatively small lymph node being involved and/or by the spread of the cancer to nearby structures or tissue.
- Stage IV cancer is extensive at the primary site, has extensively invaded the lymph nodes, or has metastasized to other parts of the body.

Staging Lymphomas

Some kinds of cancer, because of their nature, cannot be staged with the TNM system at all, or require both the TNM system and another staging method. Lymphoma is one such cancer.

A lymphoma is a cancer that develops in the lymphatic system, which is located throughout the body. There are two major types of lymphoma: *Hodgkin's disease* and *non-*

Hodgkin's lymphoma. Both can arise simultaneously in several sites within the lymphatic system, and so they are staged, as follows, by the number of such primary sites:

- Stage I is isolated to one spot.
- Stage II appears in two locations on the same side of the body.
- Stage III either involves the lymph nodes, in addition to the original lymphatic sites, or minimally involves other organs on both sides of the body (but not those that characterize stage IV).
- Stage IV has spread to the bone marrow, spleen, liver, or other parts of the body.

In general, the more cancerous sites there are, the more difficult it is to cure the disease. This is also true when symptoms such as fever, chills, night sweats, and weight loss are present. The presence or absence of these symptoms are therefore included in the staging designations for lymphoma (A-not present; B-present). For example, stage IA would indicate a lymphoma in only one location, with no fever, chills, night sweats, or weight loss.

Staging Sarcomas

Sarcomas, likewise, can arise almost anywhere in the body—in cartilage, muscle, bone, fat, or connective tissue. They are staged by the TNM system as well as by the grade determined by a pathologist. Why? Sarcomas usually do not spread to lymph nodes, and size is not quite as critical as in squamous cell carcinoma. The staging system for sarcomas is as follows:

- Stage I is a small (T1: 5 centimeters or less), low-grade (slow-growing) tumor.
- Stage II is a large (T2: greater than 5 centimeters), low-grade tumor or a small (T1), high-grade (fast-growing) tumor.
- Stage III is a large, high-grade tumor.
- Stage IV is one that has lymph node involvement (N1) or distant metastasis (M1).

Determining Prognosis

How far a cancer has advanced by the time it is diagnosed —in other words, the stage it has reached—largely determines the prognosis, or expected outcome, of the disease. The prognosis is usually stated as the likelihood that a person with cancer will survive five or more years after diagnosis. Remember, though, that a prognosis is always a generalization. Every case and every person is unique.

Finally, your underlying health and your emotional state will influence your treatment and its effectiveness. The goal of your doctors is to deliver the best possible treatment so that you live the best life possible, both physically and emotionally.

4

The Emotional Side of Cancer

A diagnosis of cancer can unleash strong and perhaps conflicting emotions. Within the first few weeks, most cancer patients are flooded with fear, anger, anxiety, and sadness. These emotions are not signs of weakness. They are normal reactions. In fact, these feelings are often so overwhelming that denial—a refusal to accept or deal with the new reality—may initially keep them at bay until the mind can gradually adjust to the news.

Everyone reacts somewhat differently to a cancer diagnosis, but acute distress is both usual and understandable. Cancer turns a person's life and expectations upside down. Emotional turmoil should be expected. However, if your emotions do not gradually ease up—and especially if they get worse—they can interfere with concentration, sleep, appetite, and your ability to follow a treatment plan or even manage normal routines. Thus they can interfere with your body's ability to heal and your mind's ability to grasp the information you will need for important decisions.

It is possible that negative emotions can impede treatment in other ways, too. Prolonged psychological stress appears to undermine the immune system. It has long been known that painful, life-changing events like divorce, the loss of a job, or a death in the family can increase a person's risk of illness. Research has attempted to explain why this happens. Some studies have shown that chronic stress can impair the ability of cells to repair themselves, a condition that clearly could influence the development and progress of cancer.

29

Other studies indicate that excessive amounts of stress-related hormones might weaken the immune system.

Coping Strategies

A cancer diagnosis, like any sudden, frightening event, can make you feel as if you have lost all control over your life. That is why it is important to identify areas in which you still can take initiative, make decisions, and exert your influence.

There are many steps you can take to ease the shock of your diagnosis and cope with the emotional turmoil it will create for a while. For example, minimizing or eliminating old and new stresses in your life will free your energies for the important challenges ahead of you. It will improve your ability to understand your illness, make informed choices about your treatment, and find new ways to care for your health and well-being. Your doctor's initial questions about your quality of life might identify "hot spots" from which unnecessary anxiety and stress are likely to arise—and there are ways of dealing with these.

Positive "Self-Talk"

Since the vast majority of cancers of the mouth and throat result from the use of tobacco, mostly smoking, many individuals feel guilty for having cancer. They believe they caused the cancer. They blame and berate themselves. Even though a cancer may have resulted from a lifestyle habit, now is a time to be loving and gentle with yourself.

If you find yourself involved with self-blame, remind yourself that you may have used tobacco for a variety of reasons, none of which included the intent to get cancer. Remind yourself that addictions are very powerful forces, and the strongest of people find them difficult to break.

Putting Yourself First

Just knowing where your emotional "hot spots" are can help you cool them down or even get rid of them. Do you find it hard to say no when you're asked for help? Do you readily take on new assignments in your work? Do you belong to clubs or organizations that hold frequent meetings and keep you out at night? Do your extracurricular activities drain you, or give you energy?

Looking at such questions is an important task early in your treatment. You must put your emotional and physical health first—before your job, your community commitments, and even many of your family responsibilities. Of course, you won't give up your family or your contacts with important groups and friends, but you can let *them* help *you* with things you have previously taken on. You probably won't give up your job, either, but you can delegate tasks, take advantage of any vacation time or sick time coming to you, and find other ways to lighten your workload.

None of this is selfish. Eliminating whatever exhausting or potentially stressful activities you can is simply necessary. In general, you should avoid tasks, people, and situations that tax your patience and energy. Seek out those that inspire you, give you strength, and make you feel good about yourself.

Reaching Out to Others

The broader your social network, the more people you will be able to draw on for strength and support. Affectionate bonds bring comfort, and they make a person feel worthwhile. Be prepared for some people to feel awkward, though. Many will not know how to talk with you about your illness, or whether they should even try. Their own fears, whether of losing you, upsetting you, or facing their own mortality, might intrude on their best intentions.

You, too, may have avoided any discussion of the topics that are now interrupting your life—topics such as illness, loss, death, or pain. So think about your relationships, and ask yourself who is most likely to help you and welcome your efforts to open up. Who is the best listener? Who knows the territory you are entering, having already been through a major illness? Whom do you trust the most? Who would help you with your daily activities, either at work or at home? Your family, friends, and coworkers will probably feel relieved and encouraged if you can tell them what you need from them.

Nutrition, Sleep, and Exercise

Good nutrition in general promotes the body's ability to heal. Plenty of sleep and rest likewise ease tension, help a person cope with emotionally difficult situations, and also give the body an opportunity to repair itself and recover from strain. Mild, regular exercise—within the bounds of your condition—stimulates the cardiovascular system and tones muscles. It also dissipates stress hormones and releases other hormones, called *endorphins,* that promote a sense of well-being. Exercising outdoors in good weather and pleasant surroundings further enhances mood.

Meditation and Relaxation

Any exercise or routine that calms the mind and creates a contemplative, relaxed mood is beneficial in emotionally difficult times. Yoga, tai chi, or any gentle, relaxed movement that stretches the muscles and soothes tension is beneficial. Deep relaxation techniques are valuable, too, especially those that focus the mind on positive thoughts or on the gradual easing of tight muscles and emotional tension. For example, meditation soothes the mind and often generates images of healing and hope. Deep, slow abdominal breathing, practiced several times a day, can sensitize you to parts of the body in which stress accumulates and can gradually help you relax them, promoting a feeling of peace. There are a great many ways to relax your mind and body. Listening to music might do it for some; painting or meditative dance might do it for others. But finding a method that works for you, one that you can sustain throughout your treatment, is one of the best things you can do for yourself.

Massages, Embraces, Pets

Any gentle contact with another warm body can work wonders in reducing distress and anxiety. A hug from a friend can ease loneliness or fears of burdening others. A shoulder rub from a mate both relieves tense muscles and communicates love. A full body massage in a spa or health club deeply relaxes the body and promotes a sense of serenity. Studies even show that having a pet, especially one that responds to caresses with affection, offers similar benefits. If you have never been a very physically expressive person, now may be the time to experience the delights of becoming one.

Getting Professional Help

What if you can't control your fearful emotions and anxieties on your own? What if your fears, depression, or anger are more powerful than all the measures you have taken to calm them? What if your family and friends, no matter how helpful, cannot meet all your emotional needs?

Every form of distress that follows a cancer diagnosis can serve a good purpose. Denial can buy you some time to adjust. Anger, especially when it is directed at the cancer, can pump you up with energy and determination. Sadness can provide release, cleansing you of tension. Even self-blame, in moderation, can give you an opportunity to assess your life honestly and forgive your all-too-human errors.

But these same emotions can become prolonged, turning destructive in the process. Denial can keep you from learning what you need to know about your cancer and its treatment. Anger can turn irrationally against your caretakers or even your family, bringing confusion and guilt. Sadness can deepen into clinical depression. And self-blame can even convince you that you deserve to have cancer.

It is vital that you talk with your doctor if your anxieties feel out of control. Any number of things can dangerously prolong the emotional difficulties caused by your diagnosis. The following are just a few situations that could call for therapy:

- You have recently suffered a serious loss, moved away from your community, or faced family or financial problems.

- You feel guilty about your cancer, either because you fear you will burden your loved ones or because you feel you caused your illness by smoking, excessive alcohol use, overwork, or other lifestyle choices.

- You encounter blaming or judgmental attitudes in others.

- You have a history of psychological difficulties, such as depression, poor self-esteem, or a tendency to avoid problems rather than facing them.

- It is your habit to "go it alone," keeping your feelings and needs bottled up when you really would feel better finding ways to express them.

Do not worry about being perceived as a complainer when you seek help for your emotional state. It is important to open up, even if you are not used to doing so, even if you have always managed your life without much help from others. If your doctor doesn't ask you the kinds of questions that will help you talk about your anxieties, you should raise them yourself or ask for a referral to a mental health professional. This is especially important if you experience any of the following:

- Anxiety attacks

- An inability to sleep, eat, or concentrate

- Persistent feelings of worthlessness

- A preoccupation with death or suicide

- A significant weight gain or weight loss

- A loss of interest in your usual activities

- A loss of interest in sex

Sometimes these are signs of a serious psychological disturbance or an undiagnosed medical condition. Sometimes they are side effects of medications. Your doctor needs to determine the underlying cause and then help you decide whether to seek professional counseling. You might choose individual psychotherapy, group therapy, a support group, or family therapy. Any of these, together or in combination, can help you improve your quality of life and your ability to cope.

Seeking therapy is not a sign of weakness, nor is a stiff upper lip always a sign of strength. When you suppress your emotions, you intensify the stress your body must absorb. When you express your feelings constructively—rather than by lashing out against yourself or others—you minimize your stress. If your relationships with others already are conflicted, so that free and honest emotional expression is hampered, therapy can often help open the channels of communication. It can also teach you how to assert yourself, look after your own interests, and participate fully in every decision you face, from treatment options to ways of handling your personal and financial affairs.

Regaining Control

The sooner you gain sufficient emotional perspective to begin learning about your illness and options, the sooner you will experience the power that information and action can impart. The more you know, the more actively you can participate in decisions affecting your treatment. Talk with your doctors. Read everything you can find about your cancer. Ask questions. Learn from other patients and survivors. As you come to understand the kind of cancer you have and your treatment options at every step, your feelings of helplessness will diminish.

Once your emotions are calmer, your stress is minimized, and those close to you are giving their support, you will be able to focus more clearly on treatment options available to you. In general, surgery, radiation, chemotherapy, or a combination will be recommended. Your doctor will advise you carefully, outlining the advantages and possible disadvantages of each possibility.

PART II

Treatment Options

Clear and Thirty-Four Degrees at 6:00 A.M. December 15

An old moon, lying akilter
among a few pale stars,
and so quiet on the road
I can hear every bone in my body
hefting some part of me
over its shoulder. Behind me,
my shadow stifles a cough
as it tries to keep up,
for I have set out fast and hard
against this silence,
filling my lungs with hope
on this, my granddaughter's
birthday, her first, and the day
of my quarterly cancer tests.

—Ted Kooser
Poet Laureate
of the United States
(2004-2005)

5

Surgery

Surgery, one of the oldest forms of cancer treatment, remains one of the most effective under the right circumstances. Doctors perform cancer surgery with the intent of removing all the cancer they can see at the time of the operation. They make these determinations by physical examination and by X-rays and scans. Most mouth and throat tumors can be treated surgically. In fact, because early detection is so common with these cancers, only 2 to 3 percent of tumors are found to be inoperable when patients are first diagnosed. Some patients, approximately 15 percent, may experience metastasis later on.

In some sites, such as the mouth, surgery is usually the preferred option. In others, such as the nasopharynx, it is seldom appropriate. The key to the decision is whether the cancer can be removed without a substantial loss of function. This is determined by weighing many factors, including the location, type, and characteristics of the tumor and the other treatment options that are available. The health professional making these determinations is a surgeon with specialized training in head and neck surgical oncology.

Removal of the Primary Cancer

The surgical removal of a cancer from its original site is known as *extirpation,* a procedure that in nearly every case takes both the cancer and a surrounding cuff of seemingly normal tissue. Usually, a pathologist examines this cuff of tissue while the patient is still under anesthesia. If microscopic analysis reveals cancerous cells, more surrounding tissue can be removed immediately. If the normal tissue does not contain cancer cells, the incision can be closed because the "surgical margins" are considered clear, meaning it is likely that all the cancer has been removed.

Removal of Lymph Nodes in the Neck

Most cancers beginning in the mouth or throat will spread first to the lymph nodes in the neck. If any nodes are diagnosed as cancerous before surgery on the primary site, they will be removed at the same time in a procedure called a *neck dissection*. Sometimes, even if no lymph node involvement has been found before the primary surgery, the surgeon may feel there is a 20 percent or greater chance that cancer could be detected in the nodes microscopically. In this case, he or she will recommend removing the nodes during the primary procedure. The nodes will then be tested for cancer, and the results will be available in two to five days. This procedure is known as *elective lymph node dissection,* and it carries a lower risk of complications than removing enlarged nodes in what is called a *therapeutic neck dissection.*

Because of its proximity to the lymph nodes in the upper neck, the submandibular salivary gland is usually removed along with the lymph nodes in a procedure called a *modified radical neck dissection,* or *selective neck dissection.* The submandibular gland produces a small portion of the total amount of saliva, and so it is usually not missed. Occasionally, in addition, the spinal access nerve (which helps in raising the shoulder) is either damaged during surgery or is removed because the cancer has spread to it.

Cancer that has spread even farther through the neck area, into certain muscles or veins, requires a *radical neck dissection,* which removes these cancerous structures in addition to the ones taken out during a selective dissection. A list of mouth and throat surgeries appears in the Appendix in the back of this book.

Possible Complications of Surgery

No matter how positive the indications for surgery, it still carries risks. Potential complications that can arise during or after surgery include bleeding and, in rare cases (less than 1 percent), heart attack, stroke, anesthetic reaction, or death. Patients occasionally develop infections, either at the incision site or in the form of pneumonia. Patients may also fail to heal, in which case additional surgery may be needed to reconstruct the affected area, or they may suffer a worsening of other health problems. Every patient has a different relative risk, depending on the extent of the cancer, the kind of operation it requires, and his or her underlying health.

Usually, the more localized the surgery, the fewer the side effects and the lower the chance of complications. Many complications soon disappear on their own. Most others can be treated successfully, often in the period immediately following surgery.

Swelling

Swelling of the mouth or throat can make breathing difficult but is treatable right away. To relieve this difficulty, a small incision is made in the lower neck, just below the Adam's apple, to create an opening to the trachea. A curved, hollow tube is then inserted through the opening and into the trachea, bypassing the swelling and allowing you to breathe easily. The opening is called a *tracheostomy*, hence the tube is called a *tracheostomy tube*.

If your surgeons believe postoperative swelling is likely, they will perform a tracheostomy during your cancer surgery, while you are still under general anesthesia. If not, it can be done later, under a local anesthetic. In either case, a tracheostomy is almost always temporary. Once the swelling is resolved—usually three to seven days after the operation—the tube is painlessly removed and the incision closes naturally in seven to ten days.

Tracheostomy tube

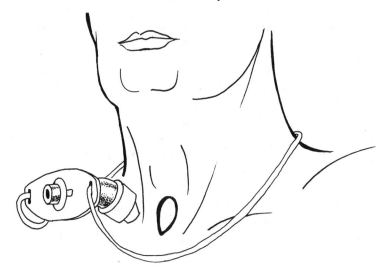

Impaired Speech

If you do need a tracheostomy tube, it might not be possible for you to speak while it is in. The tube goes below your vocal cords and diverts the air needed for speech away from them. If you plug the tube with your finger, this will force air up through your vocal cords and allow you to speak. Most tracheostomy tubes have balloonlike, air-filled reservoirs around them that allow you to be ventilated (that is, they allow your breathing to be sustained artificially during surgery), but this device also prevents air from moving into the larynx. Therefore, if you want to plug the tube so that you can talk, this balloon must first be deflated. Or, the tube may be replaced with one that has no balloon.

Once the swelling around your windpipe and vocal cords goes down, the tube can stay plugged until it is removed. In the meantime, you will be able to communicate by writing, gesturing, or pointing to special lists of common questions and phrases such as "I need to go to the bathroom." Once the tracheostomy tube is removed, usually in three to seven days, you will be able to speak normally again. The only exception, of course, is if your larynx has been removed during your surgery.

Difficulty Eating

Postsurgical swelling can also make swallowing and eating difficult or impossible. For several days or a week, until the suture lines in your mouth and throat are healed, you might receive your nutrition through a *nasogastric (NG) tube*, which runs through your nose to your esophagus and then your stomach. In most cases, once the swelling has improved and you are able to swallow, the tube will be removed at your bedside. You will be able to begin eating again.

In some patients, however, the swelling and results of surgery make eating difficult for a longer period of time. Swelling disrupts the normal rhythm of the swallowing process that propels food down into the stomach. Also, if there is significant swelling, the tongue may not move easily. It can take time to overcome some of these difficulties and relearn to swallow. Meanwhile, a *gastrostomy (G) tube*, can be placed directly into the stomach to bypass the need for swallowing. This is much more convenient than an NG tube, which interferes with speech. You or your family members will be taught how to give liquid feedings through the G tube.

The Operation

Usually, you will be asked to report to the hospital about two hours before your surgery, and you'll then be taken to the preoperative area. There you will change into a hospital gown, and nurses will start an *intravenous catheter*, or *IV*, to administer medication that will help you relax. You may not remember anything beyond this point.

From pre-op, you will be taken to the operating room. If you are still awake, you will see a machine that will monitor your heart rate and breathing. You will also see a ventilator next to the operating bed, along with tables on which surgical instruments are laid out, and bright lights overhead. The surgeons, nurses, and anesthesiologists might already be in the room, preparing for your surgery.

Once you have been moved onto the operating table, the anesthesiologist or nurse will place an oxygen mask over your mouth and nose to keep your blood rich with oxygen while you are being put under anesthesia. He or she will then administer a powerful anesthetic through your IV tube. You might feel a mild burning sensation in your arm as the medicine enters your bloodstream. When you next awake, your operation should be over.

While you are in the operating room, your family and friends will likely be waiting in a surgery waiting room. In many hospitals, a nurse from the operating room will keep family members updated on the progress of the operation. Once the operation is complete, the surgeon will meet with family and friends to inform them about the surgery.

Postoperative Care

After you awake from the anesthesia, you will be transferred from the recovery room to either the intensive care unit or the surgical ward, depending on the extent of your surgery and your overall health. You might not be fully awake or aware of what is happening until you are in your room.

How long you stay in the hospital—usually anywhere from one to ten days after surgery—will depend on the kind of surgery you have had and on your recovery rate. Various postoperative conditions can arise, some of which are matters of concern, whereas others are not. Nausea, for example, is a common, uncomfortable side effect of the drugs used during surgery, but it usually passes after twelve to twenty-four hours. The sooner you can get up and walk, the sooner the nausea will go away.

Finally, your postoperative care will include the removal of any *surgical drains*, tubes placed in your wounds during the operation to prevent unwanted fluids from accumulating. The drains are removed at the bedside after three to five days.

Pain Management

Pain management can be a more serious concern than nausea, even though surgery for cancer of the mouth or throat is usually not as painful as some other surgeries. Whatever pain you do experience can be controlled with medications, which a nurse will begin administering immediately, giving them to you on a scheduled basis if you are too groggy to ask for them. When you are awake enough, you may be able to administer your own pain medication. *Patient-controlled analgesia machines*, or *PCA*, deliver a dose of pain medication through your IV at the press of a button. The machine is set so that you won't give yourself too much. (See Chapter 10 for a more thorough discussion of pain management.)

Reconstructive Surgery

Though all forms of cancer therapy tend to cause side effects, only surgery generates the need to reconstruct or compensate for body parts that have been removed or damaged. Any cancer surgery that involves the jaw, mouth, tongue, throat, or larynx can be disfiguring and can impair speech, breathing, and eating. The goal of reconstruction is to restore these functions. Almost always, the replacement or extensive repair of structures like the jaw, cheek, floor of the mouth, or tongue are performed at the same time as the original cancer surgery.

There are two general rules for mouth and throat cancers. First, if bone is removed during cancer surgery, the major requirement at the time or later on will be reconstruction, often with little or no rehabilitation. Second, if soft tissue is removed, then reconstruction, rehabilitation, or both may be needed, depending on whether the tissue involves muscle.

Skins Grafts and Flaps

Reconstructive surgery typically uses either grafts or flaps of nonessential tissue (skin, muscle, intestine, fat, or bone) from other parts of the body to replace tissue at the site being repaired.

Skin, fat, or bone can be used for *grafts*, which do not have their own blood supply but rely on nutrients from the site to which they are moved. For example, in the case of a skin graft, the site to which it is applied will be, essentially, a fresh wound. No scars will have formed yet, so the underlying blood supply will be readily available. Usually, a very thin piece of skin is taken from the thigh to cover this site. As the grafted skin draws nutrients from the exposed undersurface of skin, it becomes permanently attached to its new site and gradually grows into a healthy, unscarred outer layer of skin. The thigh will heal with a thin layer of scar tissue.

A *flap*—whether of skin, bone, or intestine—is used in one of two ways. It either remains attached to its own blood supply (that is, it is stretched from its original site to cover an adjacent site undergoing repair), or it is removed with blood vessels attached and then, with the aid of a microscope, is "hooked up" to the vessels at the new site, creating a new blood supply.

Flaps are used more often than grafts because reconstructive surgery is usually complex enough to require an immediate supply of nutrient-rich blood. In the past, the blood supply had to come along with the flap, so only tissue from adjacent areas could be used. It had to be stretched to the damaged area. Today, microsurgical techniques and instruments allow tissue and its blood vessels to be moved from virtually any area of the body.

The kind of flap used in reconstruction depends on the kind of tissue being repaired. For example, bone flaps repair bone, and intestinal flaps repair the throat because both have a mucous lining. One kind of bone flap uses the lower leg bone (fibula), a long, small bone behind the shin bone (tibia). Because the fibula is not required for leg strength or walking, it can be removed from the leg and used to rebuild the jaw. It has its own blood supply—an artery and vein that provide its nutrients. These blood vessels are removed along with the fibula and then hooked to blood vessels in the neck near the area of the jaw being reconstructed.

Fortunately, today, postsurgical problems of the mouth or throat can be treated successfully. If patients require functional or cosmetic surgery, this is almost always done in one operation. The outcome might not restore 100 percent of a patient's original function or appearance, and physical therapy is usually required. But most people return nearly to normal.

Rehabilitation

In some cases, rehabilitation, in the form of physical therapy, can resolve functional impairments. For example, shoulder weakness, caused by damage to the spinal access nerve during a selective neck dissection, is often improved dramatically with physical therapy alone. So are other side effects of selective neck dissection, including some facial and neck numbness, impairment of tongue movement, drooping of the lower lip on the operated side, or, in rare cases, speech difficulties.

Radical neck dissection can generate more severe side effects, but some of these—such as shoulder dysfunction, or weakness and numbness caused by damage to tissues, nerves, and veins—respond well to physical therapy.

Finally, even the effects of removing the tongue or larynx can often be minimized with speech therapy and new techniques for eating and swallowing.

Restoring Speech

When cancer surgery significantly damages function or when all or most of a body structure needs to be repaired or replaced, then rehabilitation will likely follow the surgery. For instance, if the entire larynx has been removed, the throat is reconstructed at the time of surgery to create a breathing tube, or stoma. However, rehabilitation will be major in this case, since the patient must learn how to speak using one of three alternative methods taught by a speech therapist.

Electrolarynx

The simplest and most common of these methods uses an *electrolarynx*, a battery-powered device that produces sound which the mouth, lips, and tongue can form into words. The "voice" created by this device has a mechanical sound to it, but the method is so easy to use that most people prefer it to the others.

Tracheoesophageal Puncture

Another speech method requires that a small hole—a *tracheoesophageal puncture*—be made between the trachea and the esophagus, with a one-way valve inserted. This is a minor procedure, often performed on an out-patient basis. When the stoma, the breathing hole in the lower neck, is covered with a finger or valve, this forces air into the throat, which causes the walls of the throat to vibrate. The sound of the vibration can then be used to form words.

Esophageal Speech

Finally, a method called *esophageal speech* is a bit difficult to master but works very successfully for some people. The process involves swallowing air and then belching it up in a controlled fashion to vibrate the throat and produce speech. This method requires no minor surgery or devices, and it leaves the hands free. However, it can be difficult to sustain a sound long enough or at a great enough volume for good communication.

Swallowing Therapy

Patients may need to work with a speech pathologist to improve swallowing after surgery, especially if part of the voice box was removed. Here, a speech pathologist will assess the difficulty in swallowing with a modified barium swallow test. This X-ray test shows food and fluid movement during a swallow, and the various stages of swallowing may be observed. After the difficulty is pinpointed, therapies are aimed at improving the problem.

Rehabilitative Devices

For some patients, a rehabilitative device may be required when a portion of the upper jaw must be removed. Such a procedure can create a hole in a sinus cavity, which is then plugged with a special kind of denture. The denture restores the integrity of the mouth but still does not require actual rehabilitation therapy. Similarly, if your teeth have been removed, especially in combination with part of your lower jaw, implants may be considered, which attach special dentures. This would allow you to eat most types of foods and would also restore your appearance considerably.

Recovering from Surgery

Surgery requires both physical and emotional adjustments, especially if reconstruction is needed as well. During the healing phase, and after you have left the hospital, you will continue to return for follow-up visits to ensure that you are recovering well and progressing appropriately. If you require further treatment, such as radiation or chemotherapy, those issues will be discussed with you. Further treatment will begin after you have healed adequately from surgery.

6

Radiation Therapy

Almost two-thirds of people with mouth or throat cancer will receive radiation therapy. Radiation kills fast-growing cells directly or keeps them from reproducing. Cells are most vulnerable when they are dividing. If they cannot divide, they will eventually die, with no new cells to take their place.

Normal cells, too, are damaged by radiation, but they can better repair the damage, whereas cancer cells typically cannot. Some normal cells also divide rapidly and are therefore damaged more than others. This is the case with cells that make up the mucous membranes of the mouth and throat, so radiation often leads to sores in these areas. Fortunately, only those cells in the path of radiation are affected.

The strategy for using radiation will depend on the stage of the cancer and the treatment goals. For example, if at the time of surgery the cancer is found in lymph nodes or has spread beyond the lymph nodes, radiation may improve the chance of killing any residual cancer cells. Radiation therapy is also used in combination with chemotherapy, since they attack cancer cells through different mechanisms, thus potentially improving each other's effectiveness.

The decision to use radiation involves a careful weighing of the potential risks and side effects against the benefits. However, it is useful to look at one example here—a small cancer of the vocal cord. Either surgery alone or radiation alone will result in a cure in 90 percent or more of people with this kind of cancer. The advantage of surgery is that it is done in a single treatment, whereas radiation may require daily treatments over six weeks or so. However, radiation may allow the voice to recover better. Your doctor can tell you about the likely pros and cons of each treatment option available to you, and you in turn can tell your doctor which considerations matter most to you. In this manner, both you and your doctor will decide which therapy is most appropriate.

Steps Involved in Radiation Therapy

Consultation

If radiation therapy seems appropriate, you will see a *radiation oncologist*—a specialist in treating cancer with radiation. This doctor will examine you, review your medical records, and discuss with you in further detail the risks and benefits of radiation. Together, the two of you will decide whether you should proceed with this form of treatment. If you choose to do so, the next step is to determine which type of radiation to use, and for how long.

Simulation

This is the planning phase of the treatment, during which CT scans will help determine the placement of the radiation beam and the amount of radiation to be delivered, a calculation based on the size, extent, and type of cancer.

Pinpointing the tumor's location will dictate the position you will have to maintain during each radiation treatment. If you move out of position, normal cells will be targeted instead of cancer cells. For this reason, your doctors will probably make a rigid mask that will go over your face, head, and neck to hold them in exactly the right position each time. Some radiation therapists will instead place small permanent marks on your skin and use these to align your position. If you use a mask for positioning, you might experience mild to severe claustrophobia, which sedatives can relieve.

The radiation oncologist and a *physicist* will work together to plan your treatment. The physicist is trained specifically in how radiation particles interact with different types of tissues and knows exactly how to direct the machines to produce the appropriate dose and type of radiation prescribed by the radiation oncologist. They work together to deliver maximum radiation with minimum side effects. They will use the CT scans, information from your surgeon, and the results of the radiation oncologist's physical examination to arrive at this treatment plan. The plan may change during your therapy if side effects become severe.

Shields

Sometimes, healthy parts of the body are protected against the effects of radiation with shields made of a combination of lead and other alloys covered with acrylic. In particular, radiation of the head or neck raises dental concerns. Radiation reduces the amount of saliva, changes its consistency, and reduces the blood supply to the jawbone. These conditions promote tooth decay and brittleness, so a shield made by a *dental oncologist* may be used to protect key areas from radiation—especially the parotid glands, the major producers of thin, watery saliva. This allows the glands to function more normally and thus to continue protecting the teeth. The dental oncologist will also determine whether you should have preventive dental work or extractions of any non-restorable teeth before beginning radiation. This evaluation is essential. Prevention of dental problems is crucial to long-term care.

Delivery of Treatment

Both external and internal techniques are used for delivering radiation to the body. External methods aim a beam of radiation at the specific body part, while internal methods involve implanting the source of radiation inside the body.

External beam radiation—the type most commonly used against cancers of the mouth and throat—is delivered as a ray created by a machine. Treatments are usually given once and sometimes twice a day, five days a week for six or seven weeks. Each session takes place in a specially equipped room where you lie on a table and are moved into position by a technologist. Each session can last up to ten or twenty minutes, even though the actual radiation dose is delivered painlessly in just a few seconds. The extra time is often necessary to position patients correctly, especially if they are frail or weak.

A more recent technique, *intensity-modulated radiation therapy*, allows doses to be regulated very precisely for the areas undergoing treatment. The radiation is tailored to give the maximum dose of radiation to particularly high-risk areas where a tumor is present but lower doses in places that the radiation oncologist feels are unlikely to harbor any cancer. This protects normal tissues against radiation damage.

Occasionally, internal radiation, or *brachytherapy*, is used in mouth or throat cancers when a high dose of radiation to a localized site is called for. Brachytherapy involves the implanting of radioactive "seeds" directly into the body as close to the tumor as possible. For example, when a tumor is in the base of the tongue, an implant may give the highest dose of radiation with the least amount of damage to surrounding normal tissue.

Brachytherapy is used most often in cases where some cancer is still present in a single location after surgery or external radiation. Brachytherapy can be either temporary or permanent.

In temporary brachytherapy, a hollow tube, or catheter, is inserted into the treatment site under anesthetic, often at the time of the original cancer surgery if the surgeon feels cancer is still present. One to five days later, the catheter is loaded with radiation seeds. If extensive surgery was done, you will need some time to heal before they are placed. If not much healing is required, they can be loaded soon after surgery. The seeds are highly radioactive and so must be loaded in a hospital room that is equipped with lead shields. This is a painless procedure. After the radiation seeds have delivered the appropriate dose, generally in forty-eight to seventy-two hours, the catheter will be removed, usually in the patient's hospital room. While the catheter is in, however, it can transmit radiation outside the body, so contact with others is limited during this kind of treatment. This method is usually preferred for curative brachytherapy.

Permanent brachytherapy involves the surgical placement of radioactive seeds that stay in the body and gradually emit less and less radiation over weeks or months. This procedure, too, can take place during cancer surgery. It is usually performed only when the surgeon has not been able to remove all the cancer. The implanted seeds do not produce as much radiation as those used in temporary brachytherapy, so isolation is not required.

Side Effects of Radiation

Most patients are very apprehensive about side effects from radiation, which differ in their nature and severity for each person. Short-term side effects are those that last from weeks to months after radiation therapy has ended. Long-term side effects might not show up for months or years but are usually permanent. Different side effects are associated with different cancer sites.

Short-Term Side Effects

Dry Mouth

Radiation damages the glands that produce thin, watery saliva. The result is both less saliva and thick, stringy saliva, which can making swallowing difficult. Although this is often temporary, it can be permanent. If you experience this side effect, drink lots of water and also ask about salivary substitutes, toothpastes that can soothe and moisten the mouth, or medications that can help. One drug in particular, amifostine, appears to reduce mouth dryness (xerostomia) long-term if it is used during radiation therapy. Other drugs, including antihistamines, may make the dryness worse. Ask your doctor whether any of your medications will have this effect and whether you can counteract it. Also, avoid sugared or caffeinated drinks.

Mucositis and Mouth Sores

Mucositis, an inflammation of the lining of the mouth and throat caused directly by radiation damage to the normal cells, can occur ten to fourteen days after radiation therapy begins. If it becomes very painful, radiation may be delayed for a few days until it subsides. In the meantime, oral prescription pain medications, topical Xylocaine (a local anesthetic that your doctor can prescribe), and prescription mouth rinses can help.

However, commercial mouthwashes contain alcohol and can irritate the mouth and throat.

Sometimes radiation can lead to yeast infections in the mouth, which produce painful white sores requiring antifungal medications. Other sores may occur in the mouth and throat that are similar to mucositis but caused by a virus. These, too, can be quite painful and will require pain medicine or antiviral medication. Avoid spicy or rough-textured foods as well as tobacco, alcohol, and extremes of hot and cold.

Difficulty Swallowing and Loss of Taste

Not only does radiation cause mouth sores and dryness that make eating and swallowing difficult, but it also affects the taste buds so that food loses much of its appeal. All these factors can interfere with your nutrition. Some people have so much trouble eating that they must be given their nutrition through a nasogastric tube or a tube into the stomach. You can usually avoid feeding tubes by drinking plenty of fluids to ease mouth dryness and by drinking liquid dietary supplements, which provide needed calories, proteins, and vitamins. Pureed and soft foods are also fairly easy to tolerate, and dips or sauces can enhance flavor. Avoid dietetic and low-fat foods—this is not the time for them.

Since difficulty swallowing is often the most troublesome side effect of radiation, rehabilitation is frequently recommended. Here, the patient works with a speech pathologist who makes evaluations and recommendations for improving swallowing abilities. Patients who undergo chemotherapy, along with radiation, often have more swallowing difficulty that those having radiation only.

Dental Problems

Radiation reduces the production and quality of saliva, which helps clean teeth and keep them free of bacteria. Accordingly, the saliva's cavity-fighting capability is diminished. Even if you have shields to protect your salivary glands, you will need to see your dentist regularly to avoid or treat such long-term dental problems as decay, gum disease, and tooth fractures. In addition, a dental oncologist will probably recommend routine fluoride treatments to strengthen teeth and to prevent cavities.

Middle-Ear Fluid and Hearing Loss
When radiation is delivered to the nasopharynx, oropharynx, or paranasal sinuses, the swelling that results can cause fluid to accumulate in the ear and can produce associated hearing loss, which is reversible. Ear fluid often disappears on its own, though this can take months. Decongestants sometimes speed this process, or tubes may be placed in the ear to prevent fluid from accumulating. This is a simple surgical procedure, performed under local anesthesia. Only in rare cases does radiation cause permanent nerve injury, resulting in permanent hearing loss.

Eye Problems
Radiation to the nasopharynx, oropharynx, and paranasal sinuses can also damage the eyes, causing cataracts, pain in the eyeballs, or even blindness, though this is uncommon. If cataracts form, they can be removed by an ophthalmologist. It is very uncommon for the eyeball to receive extensive radiation, but if it does, blindness may occur, and removal of the eyeball may be necessary.

Skin Changes
Radiation can cause skin reactions, similar to sunburns. If radiation makes your skin red, dry, and irritated, wash only with gentle soap and lukewarm water. Check with your radiation therapist about any other skin products. Avoid sun exposure.

Fatigue
During the course of your radiation therapy, your body will be working very hard to kill the cancer cells and to heal from the effects of the treatments. Fatigue is a natural side effect of this process, though in most cases it gradually improves after treatment has ended. In the meantime, you will need much more rest and sleep than usual, and your ability to function well at work or at home may be limited. If you discuss this

likelihood with your employer and your family in advance, they will know what to expect.

Long-Term Side Effects

Bone and Tissue Injury

Radiation injuries to soft tissue and to small blood vessels to the bone can diminish the blood supply to the damaged sites and ultimately lead to permanent tissue loss. Tissue injury or tissue loss, called *soft tissue necrosis,* is usually seen in areas that have received high doses of radiation. Tissue damage will usually heal on its own but can take several months. Occasionally, flaps of tissue may be needed to replace lost tissue.

Loss of bone tissue is known as *osteoradionecrosis.* In mouth or throat cancers, the risk that radiation presents to the bones of the jaw and skull is sometimes increased by poor-fitting dentures, poor oral hygiene, and ongoing alcohol or tobacco abuse. The most likely effects are pain and exposed bone. Sometimes these will progress to complete loss of the jaw, which requires extensive reconstructive surgery.

Treatment of osteoradionecrosis includes removal of dead bone, improved oral hygiene, and possibly *hyperbaric oxygen (HBO)*—that is, oxygen delivered to the entire body under high pressure. This complex process induces new blood vessels to form, and that increases the oxygen and nutrients delivered to bone, allowing the bone to heal from injury much faster. HBO cannot restore dead bone, however. Any dead bone must be removed either before HBO begins or during the course of treatment.

HBO treatments are then given daily. Each one lasts about ninety minutes, with the patient in a small tank but able to see out. This tank is pressurized and can make you feel like you dove thirty-two to forty-five feet under water. It contains oxygen enriched air, which is forced into the tissues of your whole body. Most people manage the treatments very well, but if you have severe claustrophobia you might need medication to control it.

Chronic Skin Changes

Radiation may result in scarring of the skin and its underlying structures. This gradually turns soft, supple skin hard and "woody," sometimes permanently. It is more likely to happen if you have previously undergone surgery or chemotherapy. It is hard to predict who will have these changes in their skin. Good skin care, moisturizers, and sun avoidance can minimize these side effects, which permanently increase the risk of sunburn in the affected areas.

Decreased Thyroid Function

Radiation can permanently injure the thyroid gland, preventing or limiting its production of thyroid hormone. This hormone helps regulate the body's metabolism. It's important to have your thyroid function checked six to twelve months after your treatment ends. Fortunately, thyroid hormone can easily be replaced with medication taken once a day.

Chronic Swelling

Swelling of the neck—especially under the chin—may persist for months or years after radiation therapy. It is often worse in the morning. Usually, neck swelling resolves in six months to a year. Many patients fear that this swelling might represent a recurrent cancer, since it often doesn't show up until several months after radiation therapy and then feels like a lump under the chin. Head elevation and massage can help, but time is the best remedy. This kind of swelling usually resolves on its own.

Swelling of the larynx can affect the quality of your voice as well as create difficulty breathing. In rare instances, a tracheostomy tube (inserted in the windpipe) is necessary until the swelling resolves. This swelling often worsens right after radiation has ended, then it usually begins to resolve in four to eight weeks. Rarely, the swelling lasts for years or is permanent.

Swelling of the tongue, pharyngeal walls, palate, or uvula can impede speech and swallowing. Again, this may require a tracheostomy or feeding tube until the swelling resolves, usually in a couple of months.

Decreased Jaw Opening

Radiation scars in the jaw joint and surrounding tissues create a condition called *trismus,* an inability to open the mouth all the way. Stretching exercises can relieve this condition or, if they are started early, can even prevent it. Your dental oncologist will direct you in the proper mouth opening exercises.

Secondary Cancer Formation

A very low risk of radiation is the formation of a new cancer many years later in the site that received radiation treatment. If this should occur, the cancer will be surgically removed.

7

Chemotherapy

Even the word *chemotherapy* may raise fear and uncertainty in your mind—no doubt because its benefits have often come at the cost of serious side effects. Fortunately, in the past decade, new drugs and combinations of drugs used in chemotherapy have proven more effective in battling cancer and in reducing the severity of side effects. In fact, some of the biggest advances have been against side effects such as nausea.

Like radiation therapy, chemotherapy works against cells that reproduce fastest—cancer cells. Different drugs used in chemotherapy accomplish this in different ways. Some fool the cells into incorporating them into their DNA, which causes cell death. Others block the cell's ability to reproduce. In some cases, by using two drugs together, the advantages of each can be maximized, creating better results than either drug alone.

Chemotherapy alone is effective against some kinds of cancer, but, to be curative in cases of mouth or throat cancer, it must be used in combination with surgery or radiation. Whether you receive chemotherapy will depend on the type of cancer you have, how advanced it is, and the treatment goal. Even in cases where a cure is unlikely, chemotherapy can have palliative effects, shrinking the cancer or slowing its growth, easing pain and suffering.

Delivery of Chemotherapy

Chemotherapy drugs are usually infused directly through a catheter into a small vein, usually in the arm or hand. Some drugs are too harsh for these small veins, however. In this case, or if you need multiple treatments, several other options are available. A central venous catheter can be inserted surgically into a larger vein and left in place until your course of therapy is complete. In rare instances, the patient takes the drugs by mouth. The drugs can also be injected into the tumor and the nearby muscle or tissues, or into an artery that feeds the tumor. The latter, called *intra-arterial chemotherapy*, delivers high doses of the drugs directly to the cancer, allowing only weaker amounts to circulate to the rest of the body. This is a relatively new technique that may improve survival rates and prevent recurrence of the tumor at the original site, but these benefits have not yet been proven.

Steps Involved in Chemotherapy

Initial Consultation

If you and your doctors decide on chemotherapy, you will see a *medical oncologist*, a specialist in chemotherapy treatment. This doctor will examine you, review your medical records, and determine which drugs to use, how to deliver them, and for how long a time. He or she will review with you the risks and benefits of treatment.

Treatment

Chemotherapy can be administered in the hospital, a clinic, a doctor's office, or even in the home. It is usually done on an outpatient basis, but this depends on the drugs used and how well you tolerate them.

Duration and Frequency

Your chemotherapy treatments could be given daily, weekly, or monthly for a period up to several months. The overall plan depends on your cancer, your condition, and your tolerance for the drugs. For example, your treatment will take longer if you need extra time between sessions to recuperate from the effects of the drugs.

You might even need a break—several days or weeks off from chemotherapy—if your side effects are severe or your blood counts are low. The actual delivery of chemotherapy is not painful, though the sessions can last up to several hours. It feels like any other medication going into the vein. You may experience nausea when the drugs are delivered or soon after they are in your body.

Side Effects

When chemotherapy damages normal cells, especially those that reproduce rapidly, this causes side effects. You may experience some, all, or none of the side effects discussed below. They may be mild or severe. Most will gradually disappear after chemotherapy treatment is completed, though some can cause permanent change. Depending on the drugs used and their dosages, the effects usually intensify if chemotherapy is coupled with radiation.

The following list of side effects is derived from materials from the National Institutes of Health:

Hair Loss

Chemotherapy very commonly causes hair from all parts of the body to thin, fall out gradually, or come out in large clumps. In most cases, the hair grows back after chemotherapy, though sometimes the color or texture of the new hair is different. To take care of your hair and scalp during chemotherapy, follow these recommendations:

- Use mild shampoos.
- Use a soft hairbrush.
- Set your hair dryer on low.
- Don't use brush rollers or heated rollers to set your hair.
- Don't use hair color or permanents.
- Cut your hair short, so it will look fuller.
- Cover your scalp when you are in the sun.

If your hair thins or falls out, you might want to wear a wig, scarf, hat, or other head covering. Some cancer societies specialize in helping cancer patients with headdresses or makeup. If you plan to wear a wig, it is a good idea to purchase one before your treatments begin so you can match your hair color and texture.

Nausea and Vomiting

Chemotherapy drugs can affect the stomach lining or the area of the brain that controls vomiting. Fortunately, both nausea and vomiting are better controlled than ever by new medications. The most common antinausea medications used today include steroids, antihistamines, and others. Drugs work differently for most of us, so don't give up if one or two do not work for you. The following techniques can also help:

- Avoid large meals. Instead, eat several small meals during the day.
- Eat and drink slowly. Chew your food well.
- Nibble dry crackers or toast when you feel nauseous, unless you have mouth sores or dryness.
- Wear loose-fitting clothes.
- Avoid strong odors.
- Suck on ice chips, mints, or tart candies, unless you have mouth sores.
- Use deep breathing or other relaxation methods when you feel nauseous.

Diarrhea

Chemotherapy drugs can affect the lining of the large intestine, producing loose or watery stools. If diarrhea lasts more than twenty-four hours or is accompanied by abdominal pain or cramping, tell your doctor. Also consult your doctor before taking any over-the-counter medications. If your diarrhea persists, your doctor may prescribe medications or order intravenous fluids to guard against dehydration. You can prevent diarrhea, or ease it, in the following ways:

- Eat smaller amounts of food more often.

- Avoid foods that are high in fiber, such as raw fruits and vegetables, whole grains, beans, seeds, and nuts.
- Avoid coffee, tea, alcohol, sugar, spicy foods, and fried foods.
- Drink plenty of fluids.

Decreased Blood Counts

Chemotherapy can reduce your bone marrow's ability to make red blood cells, white blood cells, and platelets. Counts of each are likely to drop seven to fourteen days after a chemotherapy treatment. Each kind of blood cell has an important function, so when their levels drop, their function is compromised and an associated risk arises.

Anemia

A decrease in red blood cell production can lead to anemia. Red blood cells carry oxygen throughout the body, so it is not surprising that symptoms of anemia include dizziness, fatigue, and breathlessness. A healthy, well-balanced diet and iron supplements can minimize this risk. If your anemia becomes serious, you may need a blood transfusion.

Infection

White blood cells prevent infection, so when their count is low you are more susceptible to infectious diseases. There are many steps you can take to reduce your risk:

- Stay away from people with colds, the flu, or other contagious diseases.
- Wash your hands often, especially after using the bathroom.
- Keep your skin clean and smooth, so that bacteria cannot enter.
- Clean your rectal area gently but thoroughly after each bowel movement. Tell your doctor if this area becomes sore or if you have hemorrhoids.
- Avoid children or adults who have recently received vaccinations.

- Clean cuts or scrapes immediately.
- Wear gloves for gardening and housecleaning.
- Avoid tasks or tools that could cause nicks or cuts.
- Use a soft toothbrush and floss gently, so your gums don't bleed.

Although infection can involve virtually any area of your body, it arises most often in the skin, lungs, bowels, bladder, sinuses, and throat. Infections can be fatal when your white blood cell count is very low, so you should report any of the following symptoms to your doctor:

- Fever over 100 degrees F
- Chills
- Sweating
- Discomfort or burning during urination
- Severe cough or sore throat
- Unusual vaginal discharge or itching
- Redness, swelling, tenderness, or discharge, especially around a catheter, wound, incision, sore, or pimple.

Do not take aspirin or acetaminophen for any of these symptoms without first checking with your doctor.

Blood Clotting Problems

Finally, platelets—cells produced by the bone marrow—are necessary to the formation of blood clots. Thus a low platelet count makes you more susceptible to bleeding and bruising. Even a minor injury can bleed persistently or cause severe bruising. You might even develop spontaneous nosebleeds or see blood in your urine or stool. These side effects can be severe. You should notify your doctor if a nosebleed does not stop after pressure has been applied for ten to fifteen minutes or if the amount of blood in your stool or urine is large. To minimize the problems associated with poor blood clotting, take the following precautions:

- Avoid aspirin and ibuprofen, which can further impair platelet function. Always check with your doctor before taking any medication at all.

- Do not drink alcohol without first checking with your doctor.

- Brush your teeth gently with a soft brush.

- Use caution in all your activities—especially in the kitchen, bathroom, or any area where minor injuries are common.

- Blow your nose gently.

- Handle scissors, knives, and tools with extra care.

If your platelet counts become dangerously low, you will probably be given a platelet transfusion. When the count is 70,000 or higher, the risk of bleeding is low. When it falls below 20,000, the risk of spontaneous bleeding begins to increase but probably does not become severe until 10,000 or even 5,000. A transfusion is considered as a means of preventing dangerous bleeding when the platelet count is between 10,000 and 20,000. However, recent evidence indicates it may not be necessary until even as low as 5,000.

Nerve Problems

Some chemotherapy drugs affect certain nerves and can produce a variety of symptoms including hearing loss, ringing in the ears, poor balance, or numbness, burning, and tingling in the hands and feet. These effects may or may not be permanent. Use common sense. If you are having difficulty with balance:

- Be careful getting in and out of the tub or shower.

- Use the handrails on stairs.

- Use a cane if necessary.

- Avoid sharp or dangerous objects, or handle them with extra care.

- Do not wear loose or slippery shoes or sandals.

In some cases numbness goes away or becomes less severe, but not always. But most patients, even those with permanent effects of nerve damage, learn to adjust to these problems.

Mouth and Throat Sores

Chemotherapy can cause mouth dryness, irritate the tissues of the mouth and throat, or produce sores or ulcers that sometimes bleed and always carry some risk of infection. If you have sores in your mouth, ask your doctor whether medications can help. In the meantime, practice good oral hygiene:

- Try to see your dentist or dental oncologist before chemotherapy to have your teeth cleaned and any cavities filled.
- Brush and floss regularly but gently.
- Use a soft toothbrush, rinse it well, and store it in a dry place.
- Avoid commercial mouthwashes, which usually contain salt and alcohol. Ask your doctor, dentist, or nurse to recommend a mouthwash or oral care gel.

To ease the discomfort of mouth sores:

- Ask for pain medication from your doctor.
- Eat foods cold or at room temperature. (Heat can irritate sore tissues.)
- Choose soft, bland foods.
- Avoid acidic and spicy foods.

To relieve mouth dryness:

- Drink plenty of fluids.
- Moisten foods with butter or sauces.
- Suck on ice chips or hard candies.
- Use lip balm.
- Eat soft foods.

Effects on Major Organs

It is surely clear by now that chemotherapy drugs can affect virtually any part of the body—even the heart, liver, or kidneys. Blood tests are used to monitor liver and kidney function. If the tests indicate a problem with either organ, this could require a reduction in your dose of chemotherapy medication or a switch to another drug.

The heart is usually monitored by an *electrocardiogram (EKG)*, which records the heart's electrical impulses, and *echocardiogram*, which uses ultrasound to measure cardiac function. Sometimes a stress test is used to check on the heart's function during physical exertion.

If you experience any chest pain, shortness of breath, or changes in the amount or characteristics of your urine, be sure to report these to your doctor.

Skin and Nail Changes

Chemotherapy can increase the skin's sensitivity to the sun, causing rashes when you are outdoors even for short periods of time, especially in the hottest times of day. Be sure to cover up. Wear sunscreen, hats, and long-sleeved shirts. This effect is most pronounced during therapy, but it can linger for months. It is uncomfortable and annoying, even though the rashes are not dangerous. Knowing the link between sun exposure and cancer, however, it is a good idea to make sun protection a way of life.

If your fingernails change to yellow or a darker color, or if they become ridged or brittle, you can use over-the-counter nail strengtheners. Wearing gloves for household chores and gardening can also help.

Most skin changes caused by chemotherapy are temporary and fairly mild. However, more serious damage can be done if a drug leaks out of a vein during a treatment session. This can injure the skin and surrounding tissue. Be sure to tell your doctor or technician immediately if you feel pain or burning as the drugs are being administered. Also inform your doctor if you develop severe itching or rashes, if you begin wheezing, or if you have trouble breathing. These can all be signs of an allergic reaction to chemotherapy drugs.

Sexual and Reproductive Effects

Chemotherapy can affect the sexual organs, sexual function, and fertility in both men and women. Some people note an increased desire for intimacy; others find it difficult to respond sexually because of the physical and emotional stress of treatment. Good and supportive communication with your partner is most important at this time—especially if he or she is worried that intimate contact might harm you.

Infertility associated with chemotherapy can be temporary or permanent. Some men consider banking sperm before they begin their treatments. Some women who are still of childbearing age investigate the possibility of using different chemotherapy to decrease the chances of infertility. If you are thinking about becoming pregnant in the future, discuss with your doctors the chances for infertility with your particular course of treatment.

In women, reduced hormone production can produce menopause-like symptoms, including irregular menstrual periods, hot flashes, itching, burning, and vaginal dryness. Water-soluble vaginal lubricants can help, and wearing "breathable" cotton underwear can reduce the risk of infection that vaginal dryness presents.

Both men and women should use birth control during the course of chemotherapy treatments and for at least three months after completion because the drugs can be harmful to a fetus. If you think you might want a child in the future, you may wish to see a reproductive specialist.

The Importance of Support

The time you spend undergoing chemotherapy may be difficult for you and your family. The length of treatment can seem terribly long, and the side effects distressing. Do not hesitate to seek the support you need from your doctors, nurses, family, friends, a counselor, or support group. Above all, ask questions, be informed, and play an active role in your treatment.

8

Treating Mouth & Throat Cancer by Stage

For every cancer of the mouth and throat, certain therapies or combinations of therapies have proven beneficial and have become part of medical practice. Which of these therapies are used, and how, depends on the location and stage of the cancer being treated and on the patient's age and health.

Many variables affect the kind of treatment you will receive for your cancer. If you wish to be informed of and involved in the choices that go into your treatment, let your doctors know. Ask that all the options be reviewed with you so that you will understand the advantages and disadvantages.

From the physicians' standpoint, the relevant factors in any treatment are its effectiveness and your ability to withstand its likely side effects or complications. From your standpoint, you may wonder what emotional and psychological trade-offs are involved. Are you willing to undergo a high-risk treatment for a relatively small chance of recovery? Or would you rather preserve whatever quality of life is possible for you? Only you can answer such questions.

Multimodality Therapy

Surgery, radiation, and chemotherapy have long been used in the treatment of cancer, but, increasingly, they are being administered in new and varying combinations, dosages, and sequences. This fine-tuned approach is called *multimodality therapy.* A team of specialists work together, from the beginning of a patient's treatment, to consult, strategize, and deliver the

69

most promising combination of up-to-date therapies. As a result, you may not need to visit a series of doctors and undergo a range of tests before zeroing in on your best treatment options. The multimodality approach is more likely to send you directly to the specialist who can help you the most, saving not only time but considerable anxiety.

Another key issue with sometimes troubling implications is dental care. It is important to have any necessary dental work—crowns, fillings, cleaning, even extractions of non-salvageable teeth—taken care of before you begin cancer treatment. Obviously, many mouth and throat cancers develop near the teeth, which can be damaged or weakened by some therapies.

Treatment Strategies

The following sections describe in a general way the circumstances and conditions under which single therapies and multimodal therapies might be used to treat various stages of cancer. These discussions also cover some of the benefits and difficulties associated with the different forms of treatment. The chart shows the possible treatment options for the various stages of cancer of the mouth and throat.

Surgery for Early- and Late-Stage Cancer

Nearly every kind of squamous cell mouth or throat cancer can be treated with surgery alone, if it is caught and treated in the early stages, before it has grown very large or has spread beyond its original site. In most stage I and stage II cancers, surgery can often remove all cancerous tissue and thus cure the disease. (The exception is cancer of the nasopharynx, which, because of its unique location and the difficulty of removing it surgically, is better treated with radiation in the early stages.)

A few later-stage cancers—those that are small or have spread to only one lymph node in the neck (stages III and IV)—can also be treated with surgery alone. For example, in a stage III cancer on the floor of the mouth or in the nasal cavity, surgery might succeed in removing both the original cancer and any nodes to which it has spread. Occasionally, a stage IV cancer of the larynx may be treated with surgery alone, if it is fairly large but has invaded no lymph nodes at all or only one

Treatment by Stage for Mouth & Throat Cancer

	Surgery alone	Radiation alone	Surgery followed by radiation	Chemotherapy* with surgery, radiation or both
Mouth				
Lip	I ,II, III	I ,II, III	III, IV	III, IV
Tongue	I ,II, III	I ,II, III	II, III, IV	III, IV
Cheek mucosa	I ,II, III	I ,II, III	II, III, IV	III, IV
Floor of mouth	I ,II, III	I ,II, III	II, IV	III, IV
Lower gum	I ,II, III	I ,II, III	III, IV	IV
Upper gum	I ,II, III	I ,II, III	II, III, IV	III, IV
Throat				
Larynx				
Supraglottis	I ,II, III	I ,II, III	II, IV	III, IV
Glottis	I ,II, III	I ,II, III	III, IV	III, IV
Subglottis	I ,II,	I ,II, III	III, IV	III, IV
Hypopharynx	I ,II	I ,II,	II, III, IV	II, III, IV
Oropharynx	I ,II, III	I ,II, III	III, IV	III, IV
Nasopharynx		I, II		III, IV
Paranasal sinuses				
Maxillary	I, II	I, II	I, II, III, IV	III, IV
Ethmoid	I, II	I, II	I, II, III	III, IV
Nasal cavity	I, II, III, IV	I, II, III, IV	I, II, III, IV	III, IV
Salivary Gland				
High-grade	I, II	I, II	I, II, III, IV	III, IV
Low-grade	I, II		II, III, IV	III, IV

*Chemotherapy is a rapidly changing field and is often considered experimental. In the case of mouth and throat cancers, it is usually done as part of a clinical trial.

lymph node. In addition, as the chart shows, stage IV cancer of the nasal cavity can be treated with only surgery. These tumors are designated stage IV if they go through the inside of the nose to the outside, a relatively short distance and therefore easier to manage surgically.

In general, cancers caught in early stages require less extensive surgery than later cancers because they are usually smaller and have not spread to other structures. In the various mouth cancers, this can mean minimal loss of the tissues of the tongue, lip, cheek, or other structures. In cancers of the larynx, surgery can be limited to a simple excision of the cancer, to a *cordectomy* (removal of a vocal cord) or, at worst, a partial *laryngectomy* (removal of some or all of the larynx).

However, when a cancer has developed close to bone, surgery may be more invasive than when it has not. For example, when a mouth cancer is located near the jawbone but does not seem to have invaded it, part of the jawbone may still be taken out along with the cancer as a precaution against cancer recurring in the same area. In some cases only the inner aspect of the jawbone needs to be removed, making reconstruction relatively easier. The bone will be tested by the pathologist. Where bone is taken, reconstructive surgery is usually required. However, no further treatment may be needed for the cancer itself—just regular follow-up examinations to make sure it does not recur.

Radiation for Early- and Late-Stage Cancer

As with surgery alone, stage I and II cancers are the ones most commonly treated with this single therapy. Radiation alone is used when surgery (usually the preferable treatment) is too difficult to perform at the cancer site, when it would have to remove too large an amount of tissue (resulting in unacceptable functional loss), or when the patient's health is fragile. External radiation is used in such cases and can sometimes be focused on a small field, thus limiting the exposure of nearby healthy tissue and decreasing side effects. Internal radiation (brachytherapy) is usually not needed for early-stage disease.

Technically, nearly every early-stage mouth or throat cancer can be treated with radiation alone, although surgery is preferred whenever possible. In low-grade (slow-growing) salivary gland cancers, surgery alone is more effective in almost all cases. For early cancers of the nasopharynx, radiation alone is the treatment of choice, even though it must be delivered with great care to avoid vital nearby structures such as the brain, the eyes, and the nerves that supply the sensation and critical motion to the eyes.

Some stage III and even some stage IV cancers can be treated with radiation alone. This is the case if the patient cannot undergo surgery or if both the primary cancer and the sites to which it has spread are responsive to radiation. The ability of radiation to kill cancer cells and stop them from reproducing decreases as the cancer itself advances. Sometimes, however, higher doses of radiation will succeed in stage III or IV. It is more likely, however, that a combination of radiation and surgery will be required.

Combining Treatment Options

Surgery Followed by Radiation

Any cancer for which surgery is the first treatment option can require radiation as well, either immediately after the surgery or some time later. Surgery helps determine whether radiation is called for because it provides both a direct look at the tumor and the opportunity for pathological analysis. Therapy that follows another form of therapy is known as *adjuvant therapy.*

Radiation is generally recommended as a follow-up to surgery in the following instances:

- When the tumor is large (T4)
- When it is deeply invasive (especially into blood vessels or nerves)
- When a margin is positive
- When the cancer cannot be removed completely
- When more than one lymph node is cancerous
- When a single lymph node shows cancer extending outside the capsule of the node

- When the cancer is high-grade (fast-growing)—a designation used mainly for sarcomas and salivary gland cancers

These conditions are determined by the pathologist's analysis of tissue removed during surgery. In each of the situations listed above, postsurgical radiation improves, but does not guarantee, the odds that the cancer will not come back.

Although tumors tend to be larger at later stages, even small ones can be difficult to remove completely. Thus, radiation might be required to kill residual cancer cells at any stage of the disease. Again, much depends on the cancer's primary site. Cancers of the paranasal sinuses can require both surgery and radiation even in the earlier stages, whereas most other cancers of the mouth and throat tend to require this combination only at stage III or IV.

Cancer of the nasopharynx is the only mouth or throat cancer for which surgery followed by radiation is not considered a first option. In this case, surgery *alone* is not used; radiation has better results.

Radiation Followed by Surgery

Surgery may be called for when radiation alone—recommended under the conditions described above—has failed to kill all the cancer. This happens much less often than the reverse (surgery first, radiation after) because no pathological analysis is available to indicate who will benefit from post-radiation surgery. In general, surgery is used if either the primary site or the lymph nodes remain abnormal after radiation treatments have been completed, or if the cancer recurs months or years later. But the side effects of radiation can weaken patients, making them less likely candidates for surgery.

Chemotherapy with Surgery, Radiation, or Both

When surgery and radiation seem unlikely to eliminate all signs of cancer, the next consideration involves chemotherapy in combination with one or both of these treatments. This may happen in stage III and stage IV cancers, and occasionally in stage II cancers of the hypopharynx, a particularly aggressive disease.

In many cases, if not most, the chemotherapy drugs that are chosen, the ways in which they are combined with other therapies, and the order in which the therapies are given are constantly being tested and altered. For this reason, chemotherapy in mouth and throat cancers is frequently delivered through clinical trials, which are discussed in the next chapter.

At this time, there is evidence to support the use of chemotherapy in selected stage III and IV cancers of the larynx. Ongoing studies are defining the role of chemotherapy in other sites. Even the dose, type of medication used, and timing are not completely known. It is important to realize that chemotherapy alone does not cure cancers of the mouth and throat and that it must be used in combination with radiation or surgery.

Changes in Cancer Treatment

The treatment strategies covered in this chapter are subject to change all the time, as new and more sophisticated therapies and combinations become available through research and testing. With each new improvement, chances for a full recovery from cancer also improve.

As you and your doctors examine the strategies available to you, taking into account your cancer, your health, and your preferences, the process will probably lead you to one of the options discussed in this chapter. Or, it could lead you to cutting-edge treatments still being tested. The next chapter discusses the administration of experimental therapies through clinical trials.

Alternative and Complementary Therapies

Some cancer patients decide to explore therapies regarded as being outside mainstream medical practice in the West. These therapies may have benefits, but they have not undergone the same controlled and rigorous testing as standard treatments. Such alternative therapies may improve the quality of life of cancer patients; however what has not been proven, at least so far, is any ability to increase the survival rate.

Therapies such as massage, relaxation, biofeedback, acupuncture, and medication may be beneficial and have little potential to do harm. However, herbs are another matter. Many herbs contain powerful substances, none of which are regulated by the Food and Drug Administration. Accordingly, approach the use of herbs cautiously, and only after discussing the matter with your physician.

9

Clinical Trials

Cancer patients often turn to experimental therapies when standard treatments have not managed to shrink or eliminate their cancers. Essentially, all drugs introduced in the United States over the past thirty or more years were experimental at one time.

By joining research studies that use patients to test new treatments, many people turn discouragement into new hope. These studies, called *clinical trials*, are launched after new treatments have already been tested extensively in laboratories. If testing indicates that the experimental therapies appear to be at least as good as standard therapies, with the potential to be even better, testing on human subjects is then permitted. This gives patients access to the most recent and promising advances. Such treatments can include new drugs, radiation techniques, surgical approaches, combinations and sequences of treatment, even gene therapy.

However, when experimental therapies are used in cases that have previously failed to improve under standard treatment, they seldom result in a cure. Occasionally, they have dramatic, positive results, but the usual benefits are more modest. Symptoms may be eased, or the tumor may shrink or even disappear temporarily. Once in a while, a patient may be cured with experimental therapy, so hope is not irrational.

Patients are often willing to participate in the hope that the experimental therapies might help both themselves and others in the future. This is how progress is made in cancer treatment—through the knowledge gained from clinical trials and the determination of those who participate.

How Do Clinical Trials Work?

Clinical trials take place in a variety of settings. *Investigator-initiated trials* are usually conducted at universities to test therapies originated by a single researcher or team. The trials are usually small, and each represents a one-of-a-kind opportunity for patients to obtain a treatment not available through any other studies. In this type of trial, participants are generally from the local area.

Cooperative group trials are supervised by a single organization but are run at numerous cancer centers, clinics, hospitals, and even doctors' offices. Several organizations have been formed just to oversee trials of this kind. Large cooperative groups such as RTOG (Radiation Therapy Oncology Group), CALGB (Cancer and Leukemia Group B), and others exist only to test new therapies or combinations of therapies in multicenter settings. They are usually funded through the National Cancer Institutes (NCI) to compare standard and experimental treatments for common cancers. Cooperative group trials are also used to test therapies for very rare cancers. Because these trials are run at many different locations, they are able to find and treat enough test subjects to obtain reliable results.

Finally, pharmaceutical companies also sponsor clinical trials of new cancer drugs in order to satisfy Food and Drug Administration (FDA) requirements for extensive testing before the new drugs can be marketed. These *industry-based trials* are held at community cancer centers, hospitals, universities, and doctors' offices. They are similar to cooperative group trials, although usually with fewer centers conducting the research. The trials are overseen by the drug companies but the actual testing is performed by individual physicians. For example, a patient who has given his or her consent may receive an injection of a known drug in a novel manner—for example, directly into the tumor instead of into a vein. The injection will be given by the patient's own physician at the hospital, but the results will be forwarded to the sponsoring drug company for analysis.

Monitoring

Regardless of where clinical trials are held, patients interests and the need for reliable outcomes must always outweigh other priorities. Researchers sometimes stand to profit from their discoveries, either financially or professionally, and institutions likewise can have a stake in a successful trial. Thus, careful oversight is required at every step of a trial to ensure that these motives remain secondary.

The first step in a clinical trial, once laboratory testing has shown promise for a new drug or therapy, is for participating researchers and doctors to write a *protocol*, or treatment plan. This spells out exactly what therapy is going to be tested, how and in what dosages it will be delivered and monitored, how many patients will participate, how long the study will take, where it will be conducted, and which controls and safeguards will be used.

Controls are especially important. They are techniques for ensuring that test results are accurate—that the outcomes of clinical trials are truly the result of the therapy being tested and not some other factor, such as smoking or alcohol intake, exercise, or overall health.

Once a protocol has been drafted, it must be submitted to an institutional review board (IRB) for approval before the clinical trial can proceed. IRB members are usually representatives of the general public (such as clergy, teachers, lawyers, and others interested in committing large amounts of time to reviewing protocols), as well as doctors and researchers who have no personal or professional stake in the trial.

The IRB monitors the clinical trial from beginning to end to make sure that it follows strict ethical standards. These standards are outlined in part by the federal government and the international community. In turn, the FDA and the Office of Protection from Research Risks (OPRR) periodically review the conduct of the IRB. These measures ensure the quality of the testing, the welfare of participating patients, and the priorities of the researchers and doctors.

The IRB will also review the *informed consent*, a document that must be signed by every patient who takes part in the trial. It explains the nature of the study and any expected side effects, risks, health benefits, payments, or costs that might be involved. Usually the cost of the drug is covered by insurance or by the trial sponsor, but routine laboratory analysis and radiographs may not be covered.

The Phases of Clinical Trials

Clinical trials typically take place in four phases. The purpose of a Phase I trial is to determine the safest dose or delivery method for a treatment and to pay close attention to any side effects it produces. Most people who enroll in a Phase I trial have either not responded to or are unlikely to benefit from standard treatments.

A Phase II trial, conducted after the best dosage or treatment method has been determined, tests whether the new therapy is effective in decreasing the size of the cancer. Researchers hope especially to see 20 to 30 percent of participants responding favorably with tumor shrinkage or disappearance. These trials usually involve patients for whom most or all standard therapies have failed.

Once a therapy has proven effective in an acceptable percentage of cases, with acceptable side effects, it proceeds to a Phase III trial, where it is compared with standard treatments. Reliable results in Phase III require many more participants than other phases. In general, Phase III trials consist of one group to which standard therapies are given and one to which the experimental therapies are given.

To make sure the two groups can be compared equally across as many factors as possible, participants must meet detailed eligibility requirements. Some trials enroll only previously untreated patients, whereas others require patients for whom radiation and surgery have already failed. The groups are then matched for age, sex, general health status, tobacco and alcohol use, and other factors deemed important to ensuring comparable groups for study. Once patients have been selected for the trial, they are randomly assigned to either the standard or the experimental group.

Usually, the FDA approves a drug or treatment if the first three phases of clinical testing produce favorable results. However, continued testing and monitoring are required even after the therapy is in widespread use. This later testing constitutes a Phase IV trial, and it documents the new therapy's efficacy and safety in even larger groups of patients. This is needed because misleading results can arise even from large Phase III trials, and rechecking the data is a further safeguard.

Not every clinical trial will require all four phases of testing. Sometimes, a trial ends early when a treatment results in excessive side effects or when it is clearly superior or inferior to standard treatments.

Taking Part in a Clinical Trial

If you think you might be eligible for a clinical trial, your doctor can help you identify one that is appropriate for you. He or she will review with you every detail of the trial's protocol and will then ask you to sign an informed consent, which confirms your awareness of risks, benefits, procedures, and possible costs or payments to you. Before you enroll or sign the consent form, ask your doctor the following questions:

- Am I eligible for the trial? What are the criteria for joining?

- How does the new therapy being tested in the trial differ from the treatments I have already received?

- How might the new therapy improve on the standard therapies?

- What risks might arise if I participate? What benefits?

- How long will the treatment take? Will I have to be away from home?

- Will my insurance cover the full cost of tests and procedures in the trial?

Once you join a trial, your participation is voluntary at each phase. You may withdraw at any time before, during, or after receiving the experimental treatment. Whether you complete the trial or not, you will receive medical care for any problems that may result from your participation. However, you will probably be responsible for the costs of such treatment. To find out more about clinical trials, visit the Web sites listed in the Resources section in the back of this book.

Advantages of Clinical Trials

- You will receive therapy that has been tested in laboratories and appears to be at least as good as standard therapies.
- You will be among the first to receive the new therapy.
- The new therapy may succeed where standard treatments have not.
- Your responses to the new treatment will be monitored closely by doctors who specialize in cancer therapy.
- Your participation may help in the development of cancer therapies that will benefit others in the future.

Disadvantages of Clinical Trials

- The new therapy may not prove more effective than standard treatments; it could even be less effective.
- You could experience unexpected, or unexpectedly severe, side effects.
- You may be liable for costs not covered by your insurance.
- You might need to travel a significant distance to participate if the new treatment is not being tested at a location near you.

10

Pain Management

Pain is naturally one of the things that cancer patients fear the most. Fortunately, this fear is largely unwarranted. Nearly all cancer-related pain—whether from the disease itself or from surgery and other treatments—can be controlled, and nearly always by medication taken orally. If you can't take pills or liquids by mouth, other methods can be used to deliver pain medication.

Pain is complex. You may have a different kind or amount of pain than someone else with exactly the same condition. Why? Pain is always affected by many factors—not just your nerve fibers, but your past experiences with pain and your current physical and emotional state. Do not be surprised if you develop pain from several sources throughout your treatment—from the cancer itself, from mood changes, from treatment and side effects, and even from some medications.

Cancer itself causes many different kinds and degrees of pain depending on its location. Cancer treatments can cause painful side effects, some of which are obvious and will be readily anticipated—for example, pain at a surgical incision or pain from healthy tissues being damaged by radiation. Others may come as an unpleasant surprise. For example, combining radiation with surgery or chemotherapy can cause muscle scarring, which generates a dull ache associated with tensing the neck or throat.

Whether your pain comes from your cancer or your treatment, it is especially important *not* to delay pain medication.

It should always be taken at the first sign of pain because this maximizes its effectiveness. If possible, it should be taken shortly *before* the onset of pain—for instance, if you or your doctor know ahead of time that a certain activity or treatment will cause pain.

Which kind of medication is used for your pain and how it is administered will depend on what is causing it, and whether it has more than one cause. Identifying the cause of pain is greatly helped by plenty of open, detailed communication. Your doctors and nurses have many tools and techniques for managing your pain, but you need to tell them everything you can. If you think you know what is causing a particular pain, say so. Patients often have very good intuition about what is happening in their bodies.

It is also a good idea to keep a pain diary. Every day, write down everything you can about your pain—even if it is mild or only lasts a short time. Keep track of the following:

- When the pain starts
- Where it is located
- Whether it interferes with movement or function
- Whether it moves around or remains in one place
- What it feels like (sharp, dull, throbbing, achy, tingling, burning)
- Whether it is constant or intermittent
- When it is worst—at what times of day and under what conditions (for example, when you are active, when you lie down, after you have eaten, when you press on the affected area)
- Whether you are able to ease it yourself,
- How severe it is

The severity of your pain is perhaps the most important thing to communicate because it determines which category of medication your doctor will prescribe. You can describe your degree of pain very accurately. Use a scale from 1 to 10, with 1 being mild discomfort and 10 being unbearable pain. If you have trouble speaking, draw this scale on paper and circle the number between 1 and 10 that applies to your degree of pain.

Why Is Severe Pain Sometimes Not Untreated?

Given how successfully pain can be controlled, you may be surprised to learn both cancer pain and post-surgical pain are often undertreated. There are many reasons for this.

Problems Related to Patients

- Reluctance to report pain, or to feel like a "complainer"
- Desire for physicians to remain focused on treating the cancer, not just the symptoms
- Fear that pain means the cancer is getting worse
- Reluctance to take pain medication—for fear of addiction, serious side effects, or developing a tolerance that can reduce the medication's effectiveness

Problems Related to Doctors

- Lack of training in pain assessment or management
- Anxiety about controlled substances
- Fear that patients will become addicted to medication, suffer serious side effects of medication, or develop a tolerance to medication

Problems Related to the Health-Care System

- Inadequate reimbursement for pain management and medications
- Overly restrictive regulation of controlled substances
- Lack of access to a pain specialist or team

It is clear from these lists that most everyone worries about pain relief leading to addiction. However, research shows that this is unusual when pain medications are monitored carefully and used for legitimate purposes. Some patients may become temporarily dependent on a drug, but this is fairly easily managed. Doctors reduce the dosage gradually, minimizing the effects of withdrawal until the dependency is no longer a problem. Such temporary dependence is not addiction, in which one begins seeking out drugs and self-medicating.

The other common concern among patients and caregivers is a growing tolerance to medication, which would make it less effective. Again, studies show that early use of pain medications does not make it harder to relieve pain later on.

Planning for Pain Control

It is important to develop a plan for pain control from the very beginning of your diagnosis and treatment. Your doctor can help you understand what to expect in the way of pain, given your particular kind of cancer and your treatment plan. You, in turn, can give him or her detailed information about the pain as it occurs. This will determine whether your pain comes from your cancer or from the effects of treatment, and your medications will be prescribed and managed accordingly.

The constant exchange of information with your doctors is important to your chances for recovery. Patients who are well informed about pain and have good communication with their caregivers report less pain, use less medication, and leave the hospital earlier than those who do not. This could be, in part, because full information increases the efficiency and flexibility of a pain-management plan. In particular, reporting any changes in your pain allows your medications and dosages to be adjusted as soon as possible. This is your best shot at avoiding unnecessary suffering.

The following guidelines are important in any pain-control plan, but most apply primarily to postsurgical and treatment-related pain:

- Make sure you and your doctor agree about the importance of managing your pain at every phase of diagnosis and treatment. Ask about your doctor's approach to pain control.
- Describe your worries, concerns, and any pain control methods that have worked for you in the past.
- Report any pain you experience at any time. Be sure to describe the pain in detail.

- Find out whether your hospital has a specialized pain service that you can call on if your pain is not controlled by routine treatments.
- Begin taking pain medications as soon as pain begins—or sooner, if you know it is likely to happen.
- Take pain medications, or increase your dose, before engaging in activities that can worsen pain, such as walking again after surgery.

Medications for Pain

Medications that directly relieve pain are called *analgesics*. There are many kinds of analgesics, and their use is the most common method of controlling nearly every kind of pain mentioned above. In general, pain is relieved by these analgesics:

- Narcotics
- Non-narcotics
- Temporary nerve blocks

Another class of drugs—antidepressants and tranquilizers—relieves pain by easing the emotional stresses than can intensify it. These drugs also have a direct analgesic affect.

Narcotics

Narcotics are powerful drugs that work in the brain to block pain throughout the central nervous system. Narcotics such as morphine, codeine, and hydromorphone are available only by prescription and are used only for severe pain over short periods of time. For patients with severe long-term pain, combinations of therapies are used, sometimes with narcotics or injections for nerve blocks.

Side Effects

Narcotics nearly always produce drowsiness or sedation, which can actually be beneficial, for they can help you get the rest you need. Other possible side effects are constipation, itching, bladder irregularity, and nausea. Most people get used to the nausea, but if it is severe, other medications can bring it under control.

Standard Methods of Administration

Narcotics can be given in pill form or as a liquid (either orally or through a nasal or stomach tube). They can also be delivered with a patch, by injection, or through an IV tube or a small tube in the spine. A patch is especially good for providing a constant dose of medication—especially a low dose over a longer period of time—and as an alternative for people who have trouble swallowing pills or liquids.

Sometimes, narcotics can continuously relieve postsurgical pain via *PCA,* or *patient-controlled analgesia.* An IV tube is attached to a pump, which is controlled by a button that the patient can push whenever he or she has pain. The pump is regulated to limit the amount of the drug that can be administered over a period of time. This is to safeguard against overdose or addiction, but, in fact, patients often use less medication this way than with other methods of delivery.

PCA is used for postsurgical pain when it is likely to be easier and more effective than having a nurse give the narcotic. The doctor will determine this based on the patient's general health, his or her ability to follow directions, and the amount of pain that is likely to occur.

Non-Narcotics

Several common nonprescription medications are used to treat cancer-related pain. These include acetaminophen (as in Tylenol), aspirin, and ibuprofen (as in Advil and Motrin). Acetaminophen relieves pain and fever but does not reduce inflammation. Aspirin and ibuprofen, which belong to a rapidly growing category of medications called *nonsteroidal anti-inflammatory drugs (NSAIDS),* relieve all three.

Cox II inhibitors are a newer category of anti-inflammatory drugs. Celebrex is an example. These have all the same positive effects as other non-narcotic pain medications, but they tend to generate less stomach upset and fewer bleeding problems. They also may last somewhat longer. Other side effects may become apparent as they gain more widespread use.

All of these non-narcotics control pain at its source rather than through the central nervous system. However, they act more slowly than narcotics and are less powerful. They are therefore used for persistent, mild to moderate pain. Normally they can be used over long periods of time because they do not cause dependency or addiction.

Side Effects

Aspirin and NSAIDS can produce stomach upset and can also reduce the blood's clotting ability, which may result in prolonged bleeding. Both can cause inflammation and erosion of the stomach lining, especially aspirin. People preparing for surgery should not take these medications. They will be able to take acetaminophen, which has no effect on clotting, and might be able to take Cox II inhibitors, as both tend to cause fewer stomach problems.

Nerve Blocks

When severe pain is highly localized—for example, at a surgical incision—it can sometimes be controlled by temporarily blocking the nerves at the site. This is done by injecting a local anesthetic such as Xylocaine or bupivacaine. There are no significant side effects to this method, and it can reduce the need for narcotics in the short term.

Permanent nerve blocks can also be used for more chronic, or long-term, localized pain. In this case—if a pain specialist determines the procedure is appropriate—the nerve in question is injected with a local anesthetic. If that relieves the pain, the nerve can then be injected with a substance that will destroy it. This leaves the affected area numb, but it usually significantly diminishes or eliminates the pain. However, this procedure is invasive, and it carries a risk of unexpected outcomes, including no pain relief at all or even increased pain.

Tranquilizers and Antidepressants

If anxiety or depression contributes to your pain, you may be given a tranquilizer (such as Valium or Xanax) or an antidepressant (such as Prozac or Zoloft) in addition to other analgesics. The calming effects of these drugs not only can help reduce pain but also can help you sleep and function better.

A fairly old class of antidepressants called *tricyclics* are especially beneficial for patients suffering chronic pain. It is unclear exactly how they work against pain, but they seem to do so in lower doses than are needed to treat depression. They are used both alone and in combination with other medications. Side effects of all antidepressants include sedation and drowsiness. Patients can also become temporarily dependent on these drugs, meaning they would need to be tapered off the drug gradually if they chose to stop the medication. They can be given by pill, liquid, or injection.

Other Pain-Control Methods

Some cancer-related pain can be relieved by methods that do not involve medications. When pain is severe, these methods are often used along with medications, sometimes reinforcing their beneficial effects. When pain is mild or moderate, these methods can sometimes be used instead of any medication at all. Your doctor may order or recommend some of the methods mentioned here. If you embark on any others, be sure to consult with your doctor to make sure they will not interfere with any medications you are taking.

TENS Unit

Just as an injection of anesthesia can ease localized pain at the site, a *transcutaneous electrical nerve-stimulation unit (TENS)* can accomplish the same result without medication. The TENS unit is a small electrical box, about the size of a deck of cards. It blocks pain by delivering a low-level electrical current directly to the affected nerves through electrodes attached to your body. This method has very few side effects except for minor skin irritation. The only drawback is that it can lose effectiveness as your nerves adapt to it.

Physical Therapy

When muscles are damaged or weakened by surgery and other therapies, physical therapy can often do wonders to reduce pain and restore strength and flexibility. If your doctor orders physical therapy, you will be given a series of stretching and strengthening exercises to do daily, either on your own or with a physical therapist's help. You might also be instructed to apply cold packs (usually for swelling) or heat packs, either moist or dry. You will be warned against using heat on areas where you have numbness. The danger of burns is always high, especially if you use a microwave oven to warm your heat packs.

PART III

Post-Treatment
Considerations

Clear and Cool
December 2

Walking in darkness,
beneath a billion indifferent stars
at quarter to six in the morning,
the moon already down
and gone, but keeping a pale lamp burning
at the edge of the west,
my shoes too loud in the gravel
that, faintly lit, looks to be little more
than a contrail of vapor,
so thin, so insubstantial it could,
on a whim, let me drop through it
and out of the day.
But I have taught myself
to place one foot ahead of the other
in noisy confidence
as if each morning might be trusted,
as if the sounds I make might buoy me up.

—*Ted Kooser*
Poet Laureate
of the United States
(2004-2005)

11

Follow-up Care

Once your cancer treatments have ended, follow-up care is important. Depending on your type of cancer and treatment, your doctor will likely want to follow up with you on a regular basis for many years.

Doctor Visits

For the first two or three years after your treatment has ended, you will need to see your doctor every two to three months, to make sure you have no signs of a new or recurring cancer. By five years, if you have remained cancer-free, you will only need a follow-up visit once or twice a year.

If your cancer is still present, follow-up will likely take place every four to eight weeks. In this case, the major purpose is to assess pain control, help with nutrition, provide emotional support, and keep the communication channels open.

Above all, be sure to keep your scheduled follow-up appointments. Follow-up visits serve three vital purposes:

- *Early detection.* This is most important of all, since new or recurring cancers and precancerous conditions can be treated most successfully if they are caught right away.

- *Relief.* In most cases, there is no new or recurring cancer, and this good news can be a boost to the spirits.

- *Communication.* These visits are opportunities to talk with your doctor about your emotional and physical well-being, your progress with rehabilitation, and any questions you've had on your mind.

One question you might want to raise in your follow-up visits is whether your doctor can suggest ways to alleviate any remaining side effects of your treatment. New therapies are always being developed, so symptoms you were told could not be helped might become curable.

For side effects that can't be cured—including some forms of disfigurement and the need for artificial speech—you might find it helpful to talk with other patients, individually or in a support group. Or you might ask your doctor to recommend a counselor.

Remember, *any time* you have a problem or a troubling symptom, you should see your doctor immediately. Don't wait until your next scheduled appointment. This is easy to say but sometimes hard to do. Many patients feel great anxiety before a follow-up visit, worrying about the possibility of facing either a new cancer or the spread of any cancer that has remained in the body. It is true that someone who has already had cancer is at higher risk than someone who has not. Still, your risk of developing a new, *primary* cancer is about 2 to 4 percent per year, so it remains relatively unlikely that this particular fear will become reality. It is difficult to predict a rate of cancer recurrence, since it depends on the original stage and location of a cancer. The range is anywhere from 2 percent to 95 percent—not very helpful figures.

It is equally important to detect precancerous conditions so that they can be prevented from becoming full-blown cancers. Such conditions can include mouth lesions, or sore spots, called leukoplakia (white patches) and erythroplasia (red patches). Lesions can be removed in a variety of ways and the cells examined for abnormalities. Treatment depends on the results of cell analysis. For example, if *dysplastic cells* are found (that is, cells that show abnormal growth but are not yet cancerous), treatment usually requires removal with a laser, excision by knife or cautery, or the topical application of a chemotherapy medication.

If cell analysis shows an increase in *keratin* (the kind of horny tissue found in hair and nails), this, too, is a danger sign, though a mild one, which becomes cancerous less than 5 percent of the time. Depending on the location of the cells, this condition usually requires patients to quit smoking, to have dentures refitted, or to remove other irritants.

You should know which symptoms to look out for in particular. A red patch is more likely to turn cancerous than a white one. A lump of tissue is much more worrisome than a soft, flat area. But *any* abnormal growth in the mouth or neck should be checked immediately—especially any lump in the neck that develops along with a sore in the mouth. Surprisingly, pain is usually not associated with cancer in its early stages. Therefore small, painful mouth ulcers, like canker sores, are seldom malignant.

Giving Up Tobacco

Every cancer survivor worries that the disease will come back—but much can be done to minimize that worry. In the case of mouth and throat cancer, especially, there is an obvious and effective means of prevention: Quit smoking. In fact, quit using tobacco in any form.

You might already have taken this crucial step. Your doctors will have urged you to do so even before starting your treatment, both to reduce the chance of recurrence or new cancer and to minimize side effects.

However, quitting is no simple matter. No drug is more addictive than nicotine, the tobacco component that keeps people hooked. Add to that the fact that you might have started smoking decades ago. By now, you have a whole set of deep-seated habits to break—smoking to calm your nerves, smoking to relieve boredom, smoking after meals, smoking just for the pleasure of it. Perhaps your friends or spouse smoke, too, so you encounter tobacco and smoke nearly everywhere you go. Perhaps you fear that if you quit you will gain a lot of weight—though, for most cancer patients, weight gain should be a goal, not a thing to avoid. Ask yourself which of these obstacles lie in your way when you think about quitting tobacco. Then develop a strategy to minimize or overcome them.

Reexamine Risks

You already know the risks of tobacco use: heart attack, stroke, cancer, emphysema, other respiratory illnesses, and the hazards of secondary smoke for your loved ones. You have already suffered one of the most serious consequences of smoking, and there is no stronger motivation than the desire not to face that consequence again. No matter how serious or long-standing your addiction, take the matter of quitting one day—or even one hour—at a time. This way, your motivation will stay strong, and your motivation is the most important factor in quitting.

Plan for Smoking Cessation

Start by giving up tobacco for just twenty-four hours. This short time is a long step toward beating your addiction. If you can quit for just one day, you'll be able to quit for just one *more* day—and keep on doing that, one day at a time.

In the meantime, look for ways to make the challenge easier. Avoid as many "triggers" for smoking as you can—perhaps long telephone conversations, lingering over a cup of coffee, feeling stressed. If you can't avoid anxiety, try deep breathing or meditation instead of smoking. Find a partner—someone else who is quitting, with whom you can share support. Some cancer centers have smoking support groups, much like Alcoholics Anonymous, and these use both the buddy system and any necessary medical means. Above all, ask your doctor for help. He or she can prescribe medications and can help you locate support groups and other resources.

Several anti-smoking medications have recently come on the market. By now, you've surely heard of "the patch," a widely advertised and very successful means of helping people quit smoking. It uses nicotine itself to fight the nicotine addiction. The patch is worn against the skin to deliver nicotine in continuous but steadily decreasing doses over time. This allows smokers to wean themselves gradually from their need for nicotine. Nicotine gum and spray are also used for this purpose. They give a quick burst of nicotine when the urge becomes strong. The gum and patch can be obtained over the counter. The nasal and aerosol nicotine sprays require a prescription from your doctor. Sometimes patients use the patch in combination with gum or a spray, but this should be done with a doctor's supervision. Depending on how much you smoke, the cost of these useful nicotine delivery systems could be less than the cost of tobacco. In any case, over time, this approach will be far less expensive than continued tobacco use.

Some people give up tobacco with the help of a drug called *Zyban*, with the active component *bupropion*. Most patients start by taking the drug once a day for three days, then increase the dose to twice a day. They pick a quit date ten to fourteen days from the first dose. During the period before the quit date, tobacco is likely to stop tasting good, and desire for it will diminish. Sometimes, Zyban also reduces addiction symptoms. You may need to stay on this medicine for three months or more in order to stay off tobacco for good.

Many insurance companies will not pay for Zyban but will pay for the anti-depressant Wellbutrin, which also contains bupropion. Ask your doctor to prescribe whichever one is appropriate for you.

Giving Up Alcohol

Limiting alcohol intake might also reduce the risk of cancer. In general, while there is an unmistakable risk from any tobacco use at all, there is less evidence of any risk from moderate alcohol use—no more than two drinks a day. Heavy alcohol use is another matter. If you routinely consume more than five drinks per day, you should simply quit drinking. Any alcohol use in combination with tobacco is especially harmful. The combination increases the risk for cancer by forty times in heavy drinkers and smokers.

As with tobacco, the first step is a desire to quit. Alcoholics Anonymous has helped millions accomplish this challenge. If you are about to undergo surgery, or decide to quit drinking all at once, make sure your doctors are aware of your usual alcohol intake because withdrawal can produce *delirium tremens*, or *DTs*. This is a short-term condition, but it can be fatal if it is not treated with drugs that ease the withdrawal symptoms.

Even if you don't have an actual drinking problem, it is always a good idea to limit your alcohol intake after cancer treatment. One or two drinks a day is probably all right, unless your doctor recommends against it. If you are an alcoholic, or have poor nutrition or mouth sores, your doctor will probably recommend that you not use any alcohol at all.

Maintaining Nutrition

From the very beginning of their illness, many people with mouth or throat cancer find it difficult to eat or swallow because of painful tumors. In addition, the cancer increases the metabolic demands on the body, meaning that more nutrition is needed to fight the disease. Patients often lose weight and muscle mass even before treatment begins. Once it is under way, side effects can make the problem worse.

All along, your doctors will have worked with you to maintain your weight and nutrition. Once your treatment has ended, you will need to learn how to manage your diet and keep your weight up on your own. Your continued healing and good health depend on this. But if various cancer treatments have left you with little ability to taste food, or have removed or scarred parts of your mouth or throat, the formerly simple act of eating can seem an insurmountable challenge. Fortunately, there are ways to address these difficulties. In most cases, your doctor will be able to pinpoint your problem and recommend techniques that can help you eat.

Nutritional Assessment

You might need to have your nutritional level evaluated. Naturally, the first indicator is your weight. If it is 10 percent or more below your normal weight, that is cause for concern. Blood tests, too, can indicate the quality of your nutrition, by measuring levels of albumen and other proteins. And urine can be tested for nitrogen levels. Nitrogen is produced by the breakdown of protein, and in malnourished patients the protein stored in muscles will break down to meet the body's metabolic demands. This is called a "negative nitrogen balance" and is detrimental to healing. It deprives the muscles of needed fuel and can lead to a loss of muscle mass.

Once your nutrition has been evaluated, you may need to meet with a nutritionist to work out a plan for maintaining a healthy diet. This person will help you determine your caloric and protein needs and some methods for meeting them. Each day, you will need to weigh yourself, record your weight, and keep track of what you are eating and how much. You might need to take high-calorie, high-protein nutritional supplements, at least for a while. You might also need to eat smaller meals more frequently in order to take in enough nutrients without taxing your ability to eat too much food at once.

Lifelong Learning

This chapter offers only some of the information that can help you maintain a good quality of life after your treatment for mouth or throat cancer has ended. It is a starting point—but you can take it from here. Keep exploring, and keep learning. Use resources available in your community and the cancer community at large. Explore the Internet. Rely only on material that is well documented. If you don't have a computer yourself, check your local library, which is likely to have computers linked to the Internet and people who can show you how to get online and search for relevant sites. Stay in touch with your doctor, and don't stop asking questions until you get the resources you feel you need.

12

End-of-Life Issues

Death is an intensely personal and often a totally private matter. Some people never think about it or talk to others about it. Some adopt a philosophical attitude, acknowledging that death will come but preferring to deal with matters at hand. Others meditate deeply on this ultimate human reality. Regardless of their outlook, though, most people remain unprepared to face their own death—at least at first.

If you have been informed that cancer treatments can no longer help you, you will probably feel overwhelmed for a while by confusion, fear, resistance—any number of conflicting and disruptive emotions. At the same time, you will suddenly need to make decisions about every aspect of your death, from the most practical to the most spiritual. This is an enormous and painful challenge. You will need all the support that family, friends, doctors, and nurses can give you—and you will need to support many of these people in turn, as they deal with their own sorrow.

Stages of Dying

As stormy as your emotions may be, they are necessary and even predictable. Most people facing death go through several emotional phases in the process of coming to terms with dying. These stages include denial, anger, bargaining (trying to "make deals" with God or life in exchange for more time), sadness, and acceptance. The dying person is not the only one to experience these feelings. Loved ones usually share in each of them, though not necessarily at the same time. Even doctors and nurses can show signs of denial, given their strong belief in the power of treatment. They, and many others, might also be uncomfortable talking openly and honestly about death.

When other people seem awkward with you or try to bolster your spirits with false cheer, gently encourage them to acknowledge the truth. Like many people confronting death, you may find that helping others adjust will help you find peace yourself. There are several ways you can help your friends and family—for example, by accepting *their* help and gifts, by graciously expressing your gratitude, and by letting them know that you understand their fears and sadness because you feel, or have felt, the same things yourself.

Above all, you should always let others know what you need and want. The more openly you are able to communicate with everyone involved in your life and your care, the less alone you will feel, and the less like a victim of fate or of life's unfairness. The sadness that dying patients experience is often eased considerably by communication—and also by positive action and assertiveness. Take care of your affairs. Make amends with people you have hurt or offended—not by asking forgiveness, but by asking how you can best repair any damage you have done. Be straightforward. Assume control whenever you can, but allow other people their emotions and honor their desire to help.

Be aware, too, that there is a level of sadness that neither action nor conversation can soothe. This kind of sadness is the grief that arises at the prospect of leaving behind the people you love, the rewards of your life and work, the pleasures you have always enjoyed. There is no avoiding this sorrow, but the more you acknowledge it, and allow yourself to feel it, the sooner it can lead you to the final emotional stage in this process, which is acceptance.

Ironically, this stage, which finally gives comfort to the dying person, is often hardest on loved ones. They may see your acceptance as a letting go, a withdrawal from life and relationships. But you can help those close to you understand that you still care as deeply about them as ever; you are simply at peace with your condition, and you wish the same for them.

Making Arrangements

One thing you can do for yourself and those you care about is to take care of every aspect of your life and treatment that you can. Only you can know for sure what you want done about your business affairs, your treatment, your emotional and spiritual health, and the setting in which you prefer to spend your last days. Spelling out your wishes and discussing them with loved ones can provide a sense of accomplishment. It is important to keep living, even as you are dying. And nothing promotes a better quality of life than drawing closer to the people you love, protecting your interests, and relieving others of unnecessary burdens.

Advance Directives

From the beginning of your illness, you should think about conditions under which you would accept or refuse certain forms of medical care. *Advance directives* protect your wishes in this regard, whether you choose to write a living will, name someone to act as your proxy in health-care issues, or both.

A *living will* is a written document that specifies the kinds and levels of medical treatment you are willing to undergo. In most states, it must be witnessed, but it does not bind you to your decisions. You can change your mind at any time. Its purpose is to let your caregivers and family know what you want if you are unable to tell them yourself.

When you draw up a living will, you will need to take into account several kinds of treatment. Talk with family, friends, or clergy about your values, your beliefs, and your reasons for rejecting or agreeing to each kind of treatment. Be very clear about your own desires; do not just try to relieve others of emotional or financial worry.

As part of this discussion, you should decide whether you want to be treated in the hospital when you become more incapacitated. Hospitals are well designed to treat acute disease but are not as well adapted to helping people to die. You should probably consider going to the hospital only if you are not getting symptom control at home.

Once you have searched your mind and heart and are ready to write a living will, you will not need a lawyer. Simply write down, sign, and have someone witness your decisions about the following:

- Life support using respirators, dialysis machines, or other equipment.
- Cardiopulmonary resuscitation (CPR). If you decide against this, a DNR (Do Not Resuscitate) instruction will be placed on your medical chart.
- Intravenous nutrition and fluids.
- Palliative, or comfort, care. This includes pain management, antibiotics, and any other measures that can ease your body or anxieties.
- Donation of healthy organs or tissues after your death.

One of the major benefits of a living will, apart from a sense of control over your care, is to relieve your loved ones and caregivers of the very difficult responsibility of deciding these matters on your behalf, without knowing what you yourself would want.

If you decide you would like to have a relative or friend speak for you, to make sure your wishes are followed, designate that person as your *health-care proxy*. You will need to discuss this responsibility carefully with the person you choose. Find out whether he or she is willing to do this for you, then outline in detail the decisions you have made about your care. It is a good idea to have a living will as well. Once you have someone willing to serve as your health-care proxy, you will need to hire a lawyer to give that person *durable power of attorney*, which is the legal right to speak for you when you can't speak for yourself.

Memorial Services

Many dying patients find it surprisingly comforting to talk with loved ones about the kind of funeral or memorial gathering they want. Some place a great deal of importance on a final ritual. Others want to keeps things simple. Some people prefer interment. Others want to be cremated, their ashes placed in an urn for burial or scattered in a favorite spot.

Whichever form of memorial you choose, planning it can let you make some important statements. The act of selecting music and readings ahead of time is a way of communicating messages that might soothe those who will mourn you. Specifying charitable donations instead of flowers, if this is what you prefer, can give friends and family a chance to feel they are doing something concrete for you.

There is nothing at all morbid about making your final plans and requests. To the contrary, most patients feel heartened by the power these gestures carry—a power to communicate with loved ones, to share beloved music or literature, to honor lifelong values, to thank those who have given help and comfort.

Taking Care of Business

You will find you have many practical and financial details to attend to at this most difficult time of your life. You may be especially concerned not to leave your family with large medical bills to pay. Most hospitals offer help with these matters. Professionals are usually on hand to consult with you about which treatments and services are covered by private insurance, HMOs, Medicare, or Medicaid. Make a list of questions and then, accompanied by someone in your family, meet with these consultants.

You may also have, or wish to find, a personal financial adviser. Tell this person about your condition and find some time to go over all your financial affairs. Be sure to draw up a legal will with full instructions for disbursing your assets to relatives, friends, or charitable organizations. You can also designate private or last-minute bequests of special items like jewelry or heirlooms simply by listing the objects and writing down the names of those you want to leave them to.

Finally, if you have substantial assets or property and want to set up a trust or foundation to manage them, this, too, is something a financial adviser can do. If you own a business, make arrangements for its sale or for new management, and make sure the books and inventory are in order. The more of these details you attend to, the fewer tasks you will leave for your loved ones and other beneficiaries to deal with. In addition, the more you do yourself, the more certain you will be that your wishes will be carried out.

Hospice Care

Hospice is not a place but a philosophy of care for the dying. Most patients receive hospice care at home; some enter a hospital and are visited there by hospice workers. Regardless of the setting—which you should be free to choose as long as your symptoms can be managed effectively—people trained in hospice care will care for your physical, emotional, and psychological needs.

Hospice care will be provided by a team of specialists that may include your regular doctor, a religious adviser, a medical social worker, and any experts you might need to help with your hygiene, nutrition, medications, or physical therapy. Hospice volunteers are also available to provide meals, child care, respite care (so family members can take a break), transportation, and companionship.

Together, this team will help you cope emotionally, will see to your pain management, will talk with you or just sit with you at length, and will make sure you are able to locate the practical or legal resources you need. They will be your advocates as well, making sure the terms of your living will are honored. Most hospice workers, including volunteers, are caring and devoted people. You will find that they deliver invaluable comfort and services.

Dying with Dignity

Every suggestion in this chapter is offered with one overriding goal in mind, and that is to create an atmosphere in which you can accept the prospect of death and make peace both with dying and with the important people in your life. Your dignity must be upheld. You can see to that best by focusing on the qualities stressed here: assertiveness on your behalf, graciousness toward others, and an active involvement in the final details of your life. Several further resources are listed at the end of this book. They can help you with every aspect of this challenge.

The Vernal Equinox
March 20th

How important it must be
to someone
that I am alive, and walking,
and that I have written
these poems.
This morning the sun stood
right at the end of the road
and waited for me.

—Ted Kooser
Poet Laureate
of the United States
(2004-2005)

Appendix

Operations for Mouth and Throat Cancers

The operations described below are the most common ones performed for mouth and throat cancers. Higher-stage cancers often require combinations of these operations. Reconstruction operations appear at the end of this appendix.

Tongue and Floor of the Mouth

Surgery: Excision of small premalignant or malignant lesion of the tongue or floor of mouth (early stage, T1 or T2)

Description: The cancerous or precancerous tissue is removed with a cuff of normal tissue. Procedure is performed through the mouth, with either local or general anesthesia, usually on an outpatient basis or with an overnight hospital stay.

Reconstruction: Wound is closed with sutures or left open to heal.

Potential disabilities and complications: Zero to minimal long-term complications

Surgery: Partial glossectomy (hemiglossectomy)

Description: Removal of up to half the tongue muscle under general anesthesia, usually through the mouth. Recommended for T2, T3, or T4 cancers. Hospital stay is up to a week.

Reconstruction: Depending on the amount of tongue muscle removed, either closure with sutures or a skin graft or flap.

Potential disabilities and complications: Range is from minimal speech difficulties to significant speech and swallowing dysfunction.

This usually is improved with speech therapy and continued practice. Temporary tracheostomy is often required.

Surgery: Near-total or total glossectomy
Description: Removal of all or most of the tongue. Reserved for very advanced cancers that allow few or no other options. Hospital stay is a week to ten days.
Reconstruction: Tongue muscle is replaced with a flap of muscle taken from either the chest or abdomen.
Potential disabilities and complications: Extensive speech and swallowing disruption. Some improvement will occur with practice and therapy. Some people will never eat normally and require a permanent feeding tube. A tracheostomy tube is usually required as well but is usually temporary.

Mandible (lower jawbone)
Surgery: Marginal mandibulectomy
Description: If cancer is close to the mandible but has not invaded it, a portion of mandible closest to the tumor is removed, usually including some teeth. This does not disrupt the shape of the jaw. This is also done through the mouth. Hospital stay ranges from several days to over a week.
Reconstruction: If the tumor is small and on the top of the mandible, near the teeth, the soft tissues can usually be closed without any flap or graft. For larger tumors, a skin graft or flap is usually required. Any teeth taken out will usually be replaced by a denture after healing has occurred.
Potential disabilities and complications: Numbness of the lower lip and gums; gum pain; inability to wear dentures; slightly higher susceptibility to jaw fracture, both during the operation and afterwards; and bone infection.

Surgery: Segmental mandibulectomy
Description: Removal of an entire segment of the lower jaw. Done for larger tumors that invade or surround the mandible. Usually performed with major resection of tongue or floor of

the mouth. Hospital stay, a week to ten days.

Reconstruction: If the bone is removed from the anterior (front) portion of the jaw, it must be replaced with bone. Small posterior defects may need to be replaced by bone.

Potential complications: The same as for marginal mandibulectomy (above). Healing is slow, and a soft diet is required for six to eight weeks.

Hard Palate (hard portion of roof of the mouth)
Surgery: Hard palatectomy

Description: Removal of the hard palate, usually for tumors of the hard palate but sometimes as part of a maxillary sinus removal.

Reconstruction: Use of an obturator, a specialized denture that covers the hole created when the hard palate is removed. The obturator is cared for just like a regular denture. Hospital stay is usually two to five days.

Potential disabilities and complications: Speech and swallowing are impaired; the obturator helps with these problems.

Operations for Oropharynx Cancers

Tonsil
Surgery: Radical tonsillectomy

Description: Removal of the tonsil and surrounding tissue. Hospital stay is five to ten days.

Reconstruction: Depends on the depth of the resection; may require a flap for reconstruction.

Potential disabilities and complications: The wider the resection, the more likely it is that swallowing problems will arise; these are occasionally severe. Swallowing therapy may be required. Temporary tracheostomy is usually required.

Soft Palate (soft portion of roof of the mouth)
Surgery: Soft palatectomy

Description: Removal of some or all of the soft palate. Hospital stay, 2 to 10 days.

Reconstruction: Usually none at the time of resection. An obturator (see hard palate surgery, above) is used for speech and swallowing after extensive removal of the palate.

Potential disabilities and complications: Without an obturator, speech may have a nasal quality, and liquids may reflux into the nose. Tracheostomy is needed only with larger resections.

Posterior or Lateral Pharynx (back and side walls of the throat)

Surgery: Pharyngectomy

Description: Removal of the back or side walls of the throat. Sometimes done through the mouth or neck; sometimes requires splitting of the mandible and lower lip (that is, cutting the mandible in half and then plating it back together as with a jaw fracture). This is all done at the same operation. Hospital stay, seven to ten days.

Reconstruction: Skin graft or flap.

Potential disabilities and complications: Severe swallowing dysfunction, sometimes permanent; failure of the fracture to heal; a leak between the throat and the neck, called a fistula, which will heal with time and occasionally requires another operation; severe swelling of the larynx, which may respond to steroids. Tracheostomy is required but is usually temporary.

Base of the Tongue (rear portion of the tongue)

Surgery: Base of tongue resection

Description: Removal of part or all of the back part of the tongue. Hospital stay is usually four to ten days.

Reconstruction: For early-stage cancers, simple closure is adequate. Higher-stage cancers usually require a muscle flap. (See pharyngectomy, above, for complications.)

Operations for Hypopharynx Cancers

Surgery: Partial pharyngectomy

Description: Removal of part of the pharynx, leaving the larynx intact. Reserved for very small cancers and usually done through the neck. Hospital stay, five to eight days.

Reconstruction: Closure with sutures.
Potential disabilities and complications: Swallowing dysfunction and speech problems, usually mild to moderate. A tracheostomy is often needed, which may be in place for several weeks to several months and occasionally is permanent.

Surgery: Total laryngopharyngectomy
Description: Removal of much or all of the pharynx and larynx. Performed for advanced T3 and T4 hypopharyngeal cancers or those that have not responded to radiation therapy. Hospital stay, six to ten days.
Reconstruction: May require a skin or muscle flap.
Potential disabilities and complications: Loss of ability to speak and swallow, which requires therapy. (See Chapter 5 for a discussion of alternative speech methods.) A permanent breathing hole (stoma) in the lower neck, which does not permit a sense of smell. Major complications include a fistula, or leak, at the incision site. (See also laryngectomy, below.)

Operations on the Larynx

Glottis
Surgery: Micro-excision of laryngeal carcinoma
Description: With either a laser or scalpel, T1 and some T2 cancers of the vocal cords can be removed with the aid of a microscope. This is done either as an outpatient procedure or with an overnight hospital stay.
Reconstruction: None.
Potential disabilities and complications: Vocal quality may be permanently reduced if the resection is extensive. In rare cases, teeth may be chipped. In extremely rare cases, the laser can cause a fire in the airway, causing burns to the trachea.

Surgery: Vertical partial laryngectomy
Description: Removal of one vocal cord and part of the laryngeal cartilage (Adam's apple). Used for T1 and T2 glottic cancers,

even if radiation has failed. Hospital stay, five to ten days; recovery, several weeks.

Reconstruction: Muscle flaps to replace the cord, rotated at the time of surgery.

Potential disabilities and complications: Severe difficulty swallowing, which requires further surgery. Hoarseness or somewhat breathy voice quality. Tracheostomy required; in rare cases where swelling does not go down, tracheostomy is permanent.

Supraglottis

Surgery: Supraglottic laryngectomy

Description: Removal of the false vocal cords and epiglottis. The true vocal cords remain intact. Used for previously untreated early-stage cancers. Hospital stay, five to ten days.

Reconstruction: Closure with sutures.

Potential disabilities and complications: Temporary tracheostomy; in rare cases, permanent. Aspiration of food and liquids into the lungs; most patients need therapy to learn how to eat safely. In less than 5% of cases, a permanent feeding tube is required.

Larynx

Surgery: Total laryngectomy

Description: Total removal of the voice box for advanced cancers of the larynx. May require removal of the thyroid gland or lymph nodes if the cancer has spread there. Also involves placement of a temporary feeding tube through the nose and into the stomach, to allow liquid tube feedings while the wound heals. Hospital stay is usually five to ten days.

Reconstruction: With the larynx removed, the trachea (breathing tube) is sewn directly to the skin of the lower neck, creating a stoma (hole) for breathing. The esophagus (formerly attached to the larynx) is sewn to the back of the tongue, creating a tube from the mouth to the stomach.

Potential disabilities and complications: Patients must relearn to swallow and speak (see Chapter 5, under Rehabilitation and Reconstruction). The stoma does not permit a sense of smell. Major complications include fistula (leak) through the incision.

Operations for Paranasal Sinus Cancers

Nasal Cavity

Surgery: Endoscopic resection

Description: For benign tumors and biopsies, an endoscope, an instrument that allows the surgeon to see areas too inaccessible through other means, can sometimes be used to facilitate removal of nasal or sinus lesions. This is usually done in the office or as an outpatient procedure.

Reconstruction: None.

Potential disabilities and complications: In very rare cases, the procedure can injure the optic nerve and cause blindness on the operated side.

Maxillary Sinus

Surgery: Maxillectomy

Description: Removal of the maxillary sinus; necessary for most maxillary sinus cancers. Requires an incision either on the side of the nose or under the upper lip. Sometimes involves removing part of the roof of the mouth. Hospital stay is usually three to seven days.

Reconstruction: Use of an obturator (see hard palatectomy, above). A skin graft may be necessary to line the inside of the cavity.

Potential disabilities and complications: Facial numbness; facial disfigurement, requiring reconstructive surgery later on.

Ethmoid Sinus

Surgery: Ethmoidectomy, often with craniofacial resection

Description: Removal of ethmoid sinus, performed for most ethmoid sinus cancers. May involve removal of part of the cribriform plate in a procedure called a craniofacial resection. May also require removal of part of the covering of the brain (the dura), if this appears or proves cancerous. The dura can be patched at the time of surgery. Hospital stay is usually five to seven days.

Reconstruction: A local flap of tissue is used to rebuild the roof of the nose, thus separating the nasal cavity from the brain. This is done during the cancer surgery.

Potential disabilities or complications: The cerebrospinal fluid (CSF) covering the brain may leak from the nose; a drain, or spinal tap, is usually placed into the spinal canal during surgery so that the leak will stop and can seal over. CSF can become infected, causing meningitis, which is treated with antibiotics. In rare cases, swelling of the brain can cause headache or even a coma. Scarring can usually be well hidden.

Eyeball

Surgery: Orbital exenteration

Description: When the eyeball or any contents of the eye socket are cancerous, the eye may need to be removed. Hospital stay is usually three to seven days.

Reconstruction: Prosthetics specialists will create a very realistic looking eye, which will be fixed with special glue or attached to implanted magnets and pegs. Sometimes a skin or flap is used to reconstruct the area around the eye.

Potential disabilities and complications: Loss of depth perception, which requires both eyes working together. Most patients accommodate well over time without any specific therapy.

Operations for Salivary Gland Tumors

Parotid Gland

Surgery: Parotidectomy

Description: The parotid gland has two lobes, one superficial and one deep; these are separated by the nerve that controls the facial muscles. If the tumor is in the deep lobe then the entire parotid may need to be removed. The incision follows the crease in front of the ear, then curves around the earlobe and into the upper neck. Hospital stay is usually overnight.

Reconstruction: None, except in the case of permanent facial nerve paralysis. Nerve grafting may be done at the time of the operation if the facial nerve is removed. Reconstruction can improve facial dropping and eye closure.

Potential disabilities and complications: Injury to the facial nerve can weaken or paralyze facial muscles on one side of the face. Facial movement will usually return within several weeks or months. Other complications include: numbness of the earlobe, which can be permanent; hollowness of the cheek where the parotid gland was removed; drainage of saliva through the incision. Removal of the parotid gland can also cause nerves that stimulate saliva to grow into the sweat glands of the cheek skin, causing facial sweating. This is called Frey's syndrome. It is not a major problem, and it often responds to medication or even antiperspirants.

Submandibular Gland

Surgery: Submandibular gland excision

Description: Removal of the submandibular salivary gland, using an incision under the jawline. Usually an outpatient procedure.

Reconstruction: None.

Potential disabilities and complications: A slight hollowing and sharpening of the jaw line. Risk to certain nerves and their related functions, especially the nerves of the tongue and the lower lip.

Operations for Neck Tumors

Surgery: Selective, or modified, neck dissection

Description: Removal of lymph nodes along the jugular vein and under the jaw. Recommended for N0, N1 and selected N2 cancers in the neck. The submandibular gland is also removed, if nearby nodes are at risk of metastasis. Usually this is done in combination with other operations to the mouth and throat as listed above. When it is done alone, the hospital stay is two to four days.

Reconstruction: None. The incision follows a natural skin crease whenever possible.

Potential disabilities and complications: The neck is thinner at the site of the surgery, but this causes no functional impairment.

Numbness of the skin of the neck, which usually gets better over six to twelve months. Nerves of the neck are potentially at risk, along with the functions they support. These include the nerve to the lower lip, nerves to the tongue, the nerve to the vocal cord, and the nerve to the shoulder.

Surgery: Radical neck dissection
Description: This takes the selective neck dissection further, removing nodes, the sternocleidomastoid muscle, the large neck muscle that runs from behind the ear to the clavicle, the spinal accessory nerve (which supports shoulder movement), and the internal jugular vein. This procedure is used for many N2A and N3 cancers. Hospital stay is usually three to five days when done alone.
Reconstruction: Usually none.
Potential disabilities and complications: Same as for selective neck dissection, with the addition of shoulder dysfunction and more pronounced thinning of the neck. Risks to the nerves mentioned above are slightly higher.

Common Reconstructive Surgeries

Surgery: Pectoralis major myocutaneous flap
Description: Use of chest muscle and overlying skin to reconstruct surgically removed muscle, especially to the tongue. Hospital stay is usually six to ten days.
Reconstruction: The area from which the muscle and skin are taken is closed. Occasionally, if a large amount of skin has been removed with the pectoralis muscle, a skin graft will be necessary.
Potential disabilities and complications: Mild weakness of the shoulder associated with certain types of movement. Usually fairly subtle. Thinning and scarring of the chest, from removal of the flap.

Surgery: Radial forearm free flap
Description: Skin and underlying soft tissue, including fat, are

118

taken along with blood vessels (radial artery and veins). This thin, pliable flap is frequently used for the floor of the mouth. Hospital stay is usually five to eight days.

Reconstruction: The area from which the flap is taken is usually repaired with a skin graft taken from the thigh.

Potential disabilities and complications: Temporary discomfort; temporarily limited range of hand and wrist motion.

Surgery: Fibula free flap

Description: The fibula is removed and used to reconstruct the jaw. Overlying skin is often used to reconstruct soft tissue in the mouth. Hospital stay is usually seven to eleven days.

Reconstruction: If only bone is removed, the incision is simply closed. If skin is also removed, a skin graft is used.

Potential disabilities and complications: Temporary discomfort and temporary inability to bear full weight on the leg for one to threeweeks.

Surgery: Rectus abdominus free flap

Description: Removal of an abdominal muscle to help reconstruct a large area of soft tissue. Hospital stay is usually six to nine days.

Reconstruction: The wound is closed.

Potential disabilities and complications: Temporary discomfort. Possible weakness or hernia of the abdominal wall.

Surgery: Split thickness skin graft

Description: A very thin, partial layer of skin is harvested, usually from the thigh. This kind of graft is used to resurface areas where bulk is not needed. Hospital stay is dictated by the other procedures performed.

Reconstruction: None.

Potential disabilities and complications: The area from which the skin graft is taken sometimes has a different color than adjacent skin.

Resources

Support for People with Oral and Head and Neck Cancer
P.O. Box 53
Locust Valley, NY 11560
(800) 377-0928
www.spohnc.org

CancerCare Inc.
275 7th Avenue
New York, NY 10001
(800) 813-HOPE
www.cancercare.org

American Cancer Society
15999 Clifton Road NE
Atlanta, GA 30329
(800) 227-2345
www.cancer.org

Society of Otorhinolaryngology and Head-Neck Nurses
207 Downing Street
New Smyrna Beach, FL 32168
(386) 428-1695
www.sohnnurse.com

American Head and Neck Society
11300 West Olympic Boulevard, Suite 600
Los Angeles, CA 90064
(310) 437-0559
www.ahns.info

American Academy of Otolaryngology—
Head and Neck Surgery
1650 Diagonal Road
Alexandria, VA 22314
(703) 836-4444
www.entnet.org

National Hospice Organization and Palliative Care
1731 King Street, Suite 100
Alexandria, Virginia 22314
(703) 837-1500
www.nhpco.org

National Association for Home Care and Hospice
228 Seventh Street SE
Washington, DC 20003
(202) 546-4759
www.nahc.org

Association of Oncology Social Workers
100 North 20th Street, Suite 400
Philadelphia, PA 19103
(215) 599-6093
www.aosw.org

American Academy of Hospice and Palliative Medicine
4700 West Lake Avenue
Glenview, IL 60025
(847) 375-4712
www.aahpm.org

Hospice and Palliative Nurses Associaton
One Penn Center West, Suite 229
Pittsburgh, PA 15276
(412) 787-9301
www.hpna.org

Glossary

A

Acinic cell carcinoma: A malignant tumor of salivary glands occurring most commonly in the parotid gland.

Adenocarcinoma: A malignant neoplasm of epithelial cells in glandular or gland-like pattern.

Adenoid: Lymph tissue similar to tonsils located in throat behind the nasal cavity, often referred to as the pharyngeal tonsil.

Adenoidcystic carcinoma: A malignant neoplasm often occurring in the salivary glands with a proclivity to involve nerves.

Adjuvant chemotherapy: Chemotherapy used with another treatment modality to increase effectiveness of treatment.

Adjuvant radiation: Radiation used with another treatment modality (usually surgery) to increase effectiveness of treatment.

Ameloblastoma: A non-malignant tumor that arises from dental structures that has a proclivity for local recurrence.

American Joint Commission on Cancer: Commission dedicated to appropriate staging of cancer.

Anaplastic thyroid cancer: An aggressive malignant neoplasm of the thyroid gland.

Anaplastologist: Specialist who makes replacement prostheses for eyes, ears and other body parts.

Anesthesiologist: A physician who specializes in the administration of anesthesia.

Artery: Blood vessel that carries oxygenated blood to the body.

Aspiration: The inhalation of liquid, food, or other material into the windpipe and lungs.

B

Barium swallow: A study in which a radiopaque suspension is swallowed for X-ray visualization of the gastrointestinal tract.

Benign: Not cancerous or malignant.

Biopsy: Surgical removal of part or all of a mass or organ for diagnostic purposes.

Bladder: Organ that collects urine from the kidneys.

Boughies: Cylindrical, flexible instruments of various diameters used to dilate the esophagus.

Brachytherapy: Radiotherapy in which the source of irradiation is placed close to the surface of the skin or within the body.

C

Candida albicans: A fungus that is normally part of the gastrointestinal tract, but which may cause infection.

Cardiologist: Physician who specializes in diseases of the heart.

Cautery: Heating device used to stop bleeding in the operating room.

Cellulitis: Inflammation of the skin.

Central venous catheter: A catheter placed in one of the central veins (large veins near the heart) for delivery of intravenous medication or nutrients.

Cerebral spinal fluid (CSF): Fluid surrounding the brain and spinal cord.

Chemotherapy: Treatment of disease by means of chemical substances or drugs.

Cyst: Noncancerous growth, usually filled with fluid.

Computer Assisted Tomography (CT scan): A special X-ray used to evaluate organs and tissues within the body.

D

Dental oncologist: A specialist who cares for the teeth of patients with cancer to prevent dental complications from treatment.

Dura: Protective covering of the brain and spinal cord.

E

Echocardiogram: Diagnostic test using ultrasound to evaluate the heart.

Electrocardiogram: An electrical tracing of the heart's rhythm.

Electrolarynx: A handheld battery operated device that is used to create mechanical speech after removal of the voice box.

Glossary

Endocrinologist: A physician specializing in the secreting glands within the body.

ENT: A physician who specializes in diseases of the ears, nose, and throat.

Epiglottis: A leaf-shaped cartilage structure covered with mucosa just above the larynx that assists in prevention of liquid or food entering the voice box.

Epstein-Barr virus: A virus implicated in the cause of nasopharyngeal carcinoma.

Erythroplakia: A red, velvety plaque-like patch of mucous membrane which may represent malignant change.

Esophageal speech: A technique of swallowing air and then belching the air to form words.

Esophagus: The portion of the digestive tract between the throat and stomach.

Esthesioneuroblastoma: A cancer arising from the olfactory nerves in the top of the nasal cavity.

Eustachian tube: A tube leading from the middle ear to the nasopharynx.

External beam radiation: Radiotherapy in which irradiation is delivered from a source outside the body.

Extirpation: Surgical removal of diseased tissue.

F

Facial nerve: The nerve that controls the muscles of facial expression.

False vocal cords: Paired structures within the voice box just below the true vocal cords.

Fibula: The outer and smaller of the two bones of the leg.

Fine needle aspiration (FNA): Needle biopsy of tissue or organ for diagnostic purposes.

Flap: Surgical creation of a segment of tissue with intact blood supply for movement to another area of the body.

Foley catheter: Plastic tube inserted into the bladder through the urethra to empty the bladder.

Follicular thyroid cancer: Malignant neoplasm of the thyroid gland arising from follicular cells within the gland.

Free flap: A segment of tissue transferred to another part of the body with microvascular connection of the blood vessels.

Frey's syndrome: A complication that can occur after surgical removal of the parotid gland characterized by sweating of the cheek skin when eating. Also known as gustatory sweating.

Frozen section: A technique of freezing tissue for examination under the microscope, usually in an attempt to determine presence or absence of disease tissue such as cancer.

G

Gastroenterologist: A physician who specializes in diseases of the gastrointestinal tract.

Gastroesophageal reflux: Regurgitation of stomach contents into the esophagus, commonly referred to as heartburn.

Gastrostomy tube: A tube surgically placed through the skin into the stomach to deliver nutrients.

General anesthesia: Anesthesia used during surgery causing the patient to be put to sleep.

Gingivitis: Inflammation of the gums.

Glottcis: Voice box, especially the true vocal chords.

Grade: Microscopic characterization of the cellular activity of a malignancy.

Graft: An unattached portion of tissue for transplantation.

H

Head/Neck Surgical Oncologist: Surgeon who specializes in the care of patients with cancers of the head and neck.

Home health nurse: Nurse who specializes in the care of patients at home.

Hospice: An institution that provides supportive and palliative care for dying patients.

Human papilloma virus (HPV): A virus implicated in causing disease including malignancy.

Hyperbaric oxygen (HBO): Treatment using high-pressure oxygen in a chamber to heal or prevent disease often resulting from irradiation.

Hyperthyroidism: A disease in which the thyroid gland produces too much thyroid hormone.

Hypoglossal nerve: Nerve that controls the movement of the tongue.

Hypothyroidism: A disease in which the thyroid gland does not produce enough thyroid hormone.

Glossary

I

Informed consent: A process in which a patient or guardian authorized specific treatment.

Institutional review board (IRB): An organization composed of physicians and others governing the implementation of studies to ensure protection of patient rights and safety.

Intensive Care Unit (ICU): Hospital area where acutely ill patients go to recover after major surgery.

Internal jugular vein: Large vein that carries blood to the heart.

International Union Against Cancer: International organization for staging cancer.

Intravenous catheter (IV): A small catheter placed into a vein to deliver intravenous fluid, medication, chemical substances or nutrients.

Inverted papilloma: A benign tumor of the nose or sinuses that is locally destructive and in 10% of cases may harbor malignancy.

L

Larynx: Voice box.

Leukoplakia: White plaquelike patches of mucosa that may be precancerous.

Lidocaine: Medication used to anesthetize (numb) tissue.

Lingual nerve: Nerve that controls sensation to the tongue.

Living will: Document explaining a patient's wishes for the use of life-support measures in case he/she is incapacitated.

Local anesthesia: Injection of medicine into an area, numbing it to pain so a surgeon can perform local surgery.

Lymph node: Small bean-shaped structures throughout the body that fight infection.

Lymphatics: Channels throughout the body that transport lymph fluid.

Lymphoepithelial cancer: A malignancy of epithelial cell origin involving lymphoid tissues of the tonsils and nasopharynx.

Lymphoma: Malignant neoplasm of lymph tissue.

M

Magnetic resonance imaging (MRI): Highly specialized x-ray using electrons to take detailed pictures of organs and tissues.

Malignant: A neoplasm capable of local invasion, destructive growth and metastasis.

Mandible: Lower jawbone.

Marginal mandibulectomy: Partial removal of lower jawbone.

Maxilla: Upper jawbone.

Maxillectomy: Surgical removal of upper jawbone.

Medical Oncologist: Nonsurgeon physician who specializes in the treatment of patients with cancer.

Medullary thyroid cancer: Type of cancer of the thyroid gland.

Melanin: Dark brown to black pigment of skin.

Melanoma: Malignant neoplasm of skin arising from cells that produce melanin.

Melatonin: Hormone produced by the pineal gland.

Metastasis: The spread of malignant cells to different parts of the body.

Minor salivary glands: Microscopic glands numbering between 600 to 1000 that line the tongue, lips, palate, throat, nose, and sinuses.

Mixed tumor: The most common tumor of the salivary glands occurring most commonly in the parotid gland. Although benign, a small percentage may convert to malignancy. Also known as pleomorphic adenoma.

Modified neck dissection: Surgical procedure to remove the lymph nodes from the neck in which the technique is modified to spare one or more of the following structures: the spinal accessory nerve, the sternocleidomastoid muscle, and the internal jugular.

Mucoepidermoid carcinoma: Most common malignant tumor of the salivary glands.

Mucositis: Inflammation of the mucosa of the mouth and throat due to radiation therapy or chemotherapy, resulting in painful sores.

Myotomy: Surgical division of muscle.

N

Narcotic: A potent drug used to treat pain.

Nasogastric tube: Tube that passes through the nose into the stomach used for decompressing the stomach or feeding.

Nasopharynx: Anatomic area of the throat located directly behind the nose.

Glossary

Neck dissection: Surgical procedure to remove the lymph nodes from the neck.

O

Obturator: Denturelike prosthesis used to fill the space between the mouth and nose.

Olfactory nerve: Nerves that control smell, located at the top of the nasal cavity.

Oncologist: Physician who specializes in the care of patients with cancer.

Organ preservation: Treatment strategy aimed at preserving an important organ involved with cancer.

Osteoradionecrosis: Bone tissue death due to inadequate blood supply from irradiation.

Otolaryngologist: Physician who specializes in diseases of the ear, nose, and throat.

P

Palliation: Treatment strategy aimed at providing relief of symptoms from incurable cancer.

Papillary thyroid cancer: Most common type of malignant tumor of the thyroid gland.

Parotid gland: Largest of the salivary glands located in the cheeks just in front of the ears.

Partial laryngectomy: Partial removal of the voice box.

Patient-controlled-analgesia: Device used after surgery which allows the patients to give themselves narcotic pain medicine.

Pathologist: A physician who specializes in anatomical and microscopic examination of tissue to determine cause of disease.

Pectoralis major myocutaneous flap: Tissue including muscle and skin from the chest often used to reconstruct the areas in the head and neck after tumor removal.

Pharynx: Throat.

Pituitary gland: A gland located near the brain responsible for hormonal regulation.

Placebo effect: When a sugar pill or inactive medicine is given to a person without their knowledge that it is an inactive medicine, and they get better.

Platelets: Components circulating in the bloodstream that assist with blood clotting.

Pleomorphic adenoma: The most common tumor of the salivary glands occurring most commonly in the parotid gland. Although benign, a small percentage may convert to malignancy. Also known as a mixed tumor.

Polyp: Inflammatory mass of swollen mucosa.

Primary: Relating to the first growth or development of a tumor.

Prosthetics: Synthetic material used to replace tissue.

Prosthodontist: A specialist in the use of prosthetic medical material.

Pulse oximeter: Machine that continuously measures the level of oxygenation in the blood through a small device attached to a fingertip or earlobe.

R

Radial forearm flap: A flap of tissue from the forearm used to reconstruct surgical defects.

Radiation oncologist: A physician who specializes in the use of irradiation to treat disease, especially malignant tumors.

Radiation therapy: The use of irradiation to treat disease.

Radical neck dissection: Surgical removal of the lymph nodes in the neck along with the spinal accessory nerve, internal jugular vein and sternocleidomastoid muscle.

Radiologist: Physician trained to perform and interpret X-ray studies.

Radius: The outer of the two bones in the forearm.

Respiratory therapist: A healthcare worker with formal training in diseases of the lungs who administers treatments to hospitalized patients with lung ailments.

S

Salivary glands: Glands located in the head and neck responsible for production of saliva.

Sarcoma: Malignant tumor that arises from connective tissue, muscle, bone, or cartilage.

Scapula: Shoulder-blade bone.

Second primary: A new tumor unrelated to an original tumor, in contrast to recurrent tumor or metastasis.

Simulation: The planning phase for treatment with irradiation.

Glossary

Sinuses (ethmoid, frontal, maxillary, and sphenoid): Paired bony cavities lined by mucous membranes contiguous with the nasal cavity.

Skin graft: Skin harvested from another part of the body to resurface another area of the body.

Speech pathologist: Specialist trained to help with speech and swallowing disorders.

Spinal accessory nerve: Nerve located in the neck controlling movement of the trapezius muscle. Injury to this nerve can result in difficulty elevating the shoulder.

Squamous cell carcinoma: Malignant neoplasm arising from epithelial cells, and the most common malignant tumor of the head and neck.

Staging: Process of how advanced a malignant neoplasm is determined.

Sternocleidomastoid muscle: Large muscle within the neck extending from behind the ear to the middle of the base of the neck.

Stoma: Opening between the skin and windpipe.

Subglottis: Area of the airway located just below the vocal cords.

Sublingual gland: Salivary gland located on the inside of the mouth between the side of the tongue and the jawbone.

Submandibular gland: Salivary gland located just below and near the jawbone.

Supraglottic laryngectomy: Removal of the top portion of the voice box.

Supraglottis: Area of the airway located just above the vocal cords.

T

TNM system: A staging system used to assess how advanced a neoplasm is including size of the tumor, presence of spread to lymph nodes, and metastasis.

Thrush: Fungal infection of the mouth or throat.

Thyroid gland: Gland in the neck under the Adam's apple that secretes thyroid hormone.

Thyroid hormone: Hormone secreted by the thyroid gland that helps regulate the body's metabolism.

Thyroid stimulating hormone: Hormone secreted by the pituitary gland that regulates the production of thyroid hormone.

Thyroidectomy: Surgical removal of the thyroid gland.

Total laryngectomy: Surgical removal of the entire voice box.

Tracheoesophageal puncture: A surgical communication created between the trachea (windpipe) and esophagus where a valve is placed so that air can be shunted to the esophagus and then belched to form speech.

Tracheostomy: Surgical creation of a hole in the windpipe to assist with breathing.

Trapezius muscle: Large muscle on the back of the neck, shoulder, and upper back that assists with elevation of the shoulder.

Trismus: Limited opening of the jaws.

Tumor: Swelling or mass of tissue synonymous with neoplasm.

U

Ultrasound: Diagnostic test that uses sound waves to evaluate tissues and organs.

V

Vocal cords: Paired cords of tissue within the voice box that vibrate to produce speech.

X

Xerostomia: Dry mouth.

Index

A

acinic cell carcinoma, 127
adenocarcinoma, 13, 127
adenoid, 7, 13–14, 127
adenoid cystic carcinoma, 12–13, 127
adjuvant chemotherapy, 127
adjuvant radiation, 127
adjuvant therapy, 74
advanced directive, 104–105
alcohol, 4, 99–100
alternative therapy, 77
ameloblastoma, 127
American Joint Commission on Cancer, 127
analgesics, 88
anaplastic thyroid cancer, 127
anaplastologist, 127
anemia, 6, 64
anesthesia, 21, 42, 56, 111, 129–131
anesthesiologist, 43, 127
arrangements prior to death, 104–107
artery, 46, 61, 121, 127
aspiration, 17, 116, 127
asymmetry, 18

B

barium swallow, 48, 127
base of tongue resection, 114
benign tumor, 3, 12, 16–17, 127
biopsy, 20–21, 23, 27, 127–128
bladder, 4, 65, 88, 128
blood clotting, 65–66
blood count, 64
Bloom's syndrome, 5
bone flap, 46
bone injury, 57–58
boughies, 128
brachytherapy, 53–54, 128
bupivacaine, 90
bupropion, 99

C

CALGB (Cancer and Leukemia Group B), 79
cancer, 1–3. *See also* specific types of
candida albicans, 128
carcinoma, 12–13. *See also* specific types of
cardiologist, 128
cardiopulmonary resuscitation (CPR), 105
catheter. *See* specific types of

Index

sunlight, 5
supraglottic laryngectomy, 116, 134
supraglottis, 8, 72, 116, 134
surgery, 43–45. *See also* specific cancers; specific types of
  chemotherapy with, 72, 76
  complications of, possible, 41–43
  followed by radiation therapy/treatment, 74–75
  radiation treatment/therapy followed by, 75–76
  reconstructive, 45–46, 120–121
  recovering from, 49
  rehabilitation following, 46–48
  speech restoration following, 47–48
  swallowing therapy following, 48
  tracheostomy tube and, 42, 112–116
surgical drain, 44
swallowing, 17, 48, 55–56
swelling, 41–42, 58–59

T

taste, loss of, 55–56
team approach to diagnosis, 23–24
temporary brachytherapy, 53–54
temporary tracheostomy tube, 42
therapeutic neck dissection, 40
therapy. *See* specific types of
throat, 6, 16, 67. *See also* pharynx
thrush, 134
thyroid gland, 20, 58, 116, 134
thyroid gland cancer. *See* specific types of

thyroid hormone, 58, 134
thyroid stimulating hormone, 134
thyroidectomy, 134
tibia, 46
tissue injury, 57–58
TNM system, 25–28, 134
tobacco, 3–4, 97–99
tongue and floor of mouth surgery, 111–112
tonsillectomy, 113
tonsils, 113
total glossectomy, 112
total laryngectomy, 116, 134
total laryngopharyngectomy, 115
tracheoesophageal puncture, 47–48, 134–135
tracheostomy tube, 41–42, 112–116, 135
transcutaneous electrical nerve-stimulation unit (TENS), 91
trapezius muscle, 10, 135
tricyclics, 91
trismus, 59, 135
true vocal cords, 8, 116
tumor, 21, 25–26. *See also* specific types of

U

ultrasound, 23, 68, 135
uvula, 7

V

Valium, 90
vertical partial laryngectomy, 115–116
vocal cords, 8, 16, 20, 115–116, 135
vomiting, 63

X

X-ray, 21–22

Index

Xanax, 90
Xeroderma pigmentosum, 6
xerostomia, 54, 135
Xylocaine, 90
Z
Zoloft, 91
Zyban, 99

About the Authors

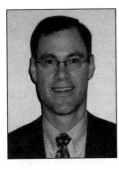 **William Lydiatt, M.D.,** is a board-certified otolaryngologist—head and neck surgeon. He practices oncology surgery at the University of Nebraska Medical Center, Nebraska Methodist Hospital, and Veteran's Administration Medical Center in Omaha, Nebraska. He also teaches and performs research at the University of Nebraska School of Medicine. His research interests include the prevention of cancer and improving the quality of life for head and neck cancer patients.

Dr. Lydiatt received his undergraduate degree in biology from Stanford University, then his medical degree and residency training in otolaryngology—head and neck surgery—from the University of Nebraska. He also completed a two-year fellowship in head and neck surgical oncology at Memorial Sloan-Kettering Cancer Center in New York City.

Dr. Lydiatt is a fellow of the American College of Surgeons, American Academy of Otolaryngology—Head and Neck Surgery, and American Head and Neck Society. He serves on the American Joint Commission on Cancer Staging Subcommittee for head and neck cancer staging; he is a reviewer for six specialty journals. Dr. Lydiatt has authored thirty scientific publications and given dozens of local, national, and international presentations on head and neck cancer.

Dr. Lydiatt and his wife, Kathy, have three children—Max, Joe, and Samantha.

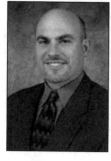

Perry Johnson, M.D., F.A.C.S., is a board-certified plastic and reconstructive surgeon. He is also board-certified in otolaryngology—head and neck surgery. He practices at the University of Nebraska Medical Center in Omaha, Nebraska. His areas of interest and expertise include reconstruction after head and neck cancer and breast cancer. He also has a strong interest in the rehabilitation of patients with facial nerve paralysis.

Dr. Johnson received his undergraduate degree in chemistry from the University of Kansas. He also received his medical degree at the University of Kansas. Following medical school he completed a residency in otolaryngology—head and neck surgery—at the University of Nebraska. He also completed a residency in plastic and reconstructive surgery at the University of Pittsburgh.

Dr. Johnson is a Fellow of the American College of Surgeons, American Society of Plastic Surgeons, American Academy of Otolaryngology—Head and Neck Surgery, American Academy of Facial Plastic and Reconstructive Surgery, and the American Medical Association. He also serves on the editorial board of Archives of Facial Plastic Surgery. Dr. Johnson has authored twenty scientific publications and has presented nationally and internationally on topics of plastic and reconstructive surgery.

Dr. Johnson and his wife Ann have three children—Taylor, Kaitlin, and Rachel.

Consumer Health Titles from Addicus Books

Visit our online catalog at www.AddicusBooks.com

To Order Books:
Visit us online at: www.AddicusBooks.com
Call toll free: (800) 888-4741

For discounts on bulk purchases, call our Special Sales
Department at (402) 330-7493.
Or email us at: info@Addicus Books.com

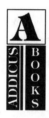

Addicus Books
P. O. Box 45327
Omaha, NE 68145

*Addicus Books is dedicated to publishing consumer health books
that comfort and educate.*